Lipidology a Primer

THE WHAT, WHY, AND HOW OF BETTER LIPID MANAGEMENT

Robert Gleeson, MD, FACP, FNLA
Fellow American Board of Clinical Lipidology
Michael Davidson, MD, FNLA, FACC
Fellow American Board of Clinical Lipidology

Lipidology, A Primer: the what, why, and how of better lipid management, second edition
By Robert Gleeson and Michael Davidson
Published by Prevent CVD, LLC

ISBN 978-0-9844225-3-1 0-9844225-3-6

Please address all requests and permissions to

Dr. Robert Gleeson
Prevent CVD Publishing
9705 North Lake Drive
Milwaukee, WI 53217-6103

Or

amanda.preventcvd@gmail.com

Illustrations and charts by RADesmarais
Interior and Cover Design by 1106 Design at 1106design.com

Printed in the United States using Goudy Old Style BT.

Lipidology, A Primer: The What, Why and How of Better Lipid Management is an introduction to lipids, lipoproteins, and lipid management. The purpose of this book is to provide basic information on lipid science and treatment. Information on best practices is changing rapidly based on ongoing scientific data and research.

This book is a guide to treatment. Final decisions on patient management are the responsibility of the patient's physician or provider and need to be individualized to each patient. All patients have individual needs that must be considered in the totality of their medical care.

The provider should always check with and follow the most current official guidelines published by the National Cholesterol Education Program, the American Heart Association, the American Diabetes Association, and other authoritative associations. The provider should always check the FDA-approved prescribing information for each drug before using that drug in a patient.

Errors of omission or commission are not intentional. If you find errors or have suggestions for improvement, please forward them to *robertgleeson@preventcvd-publishing.com*. Readers of the next edition and I thank you.

Publisher's Cataloging-in-Publication
(Provided by Quality Books, Inc.)

Gleeson, Robert.
Lipidology, a primer : the what, why and how of better lipid management / by Robert Gleeson and Michael Davidson.—1st ed.
p. cm.
Includes bibliographical references and index.
ISBN– 978-0-9844225-3-1
ISBN– 0-9844225-3-6

1. Lipids—Metabolism—Disorders—Treatment.
I. Davidson, Michael, 1956– II. Title.

RC632.L5G54 2010 616.3'99706
QBI10-600149

Author's note

We wrote *Lipidology, a Primer* for you. We wanted to fill the knowledge gap between the lipid experts, who increasingly talk with each other at the PhD level, and you, who while left out of these conversations, struggle to provide the best-quality lipid management for your patients.

Writing this text, we had three goals: (1) to help you better lower the risk of cardiovascular disease in your lipid patients and (2) to teach you as much lipidology as we could while (3) keeping the book both short and readable. To accomplish this, we had to sacrifice some scientific precision for the sake of readability.

If you want more information, we encourage you to join the National Lipid Association (www.lipid.org), read some of the excellent lipid texts they list under references (this text is listed there in the interest of full disclosure), attend their conferences, and then study for the boards in lipidology.

We hope this book serves its purpose and that you stay interested in lipid management. Our shared goal is to further prevent the heavy burden of cardiovascular disease.

Lower lipids, live longer.

Robert Gleeson and Michael Davidson

Preface

The What, Why, and How of Better Lipid Management

We wrote this book for all practitioners who want to reduce the risk of premature cardio-vascular disease, who want to better treat their difficult patients, and who want to know why they should treat their patients this way and not that way.

All too often, lipid abnormalities are treated only after clinical disease is diagnosed or they are inadequately treated. Our shared task is to treat lipid abnormalities with the goal of preventing cardiovascular disease and premature death.

We are firmly convinced that by working together toward scientifically supported lipid and prevention goals, we can further reduce the risk of cardiovascular disease. We wrote this text to increase your understanding of lipid science and your awareness of specific lipid disorders, and to improve your ability to treat your patients to lower their risk of future disease.

This text is not meant to be a definitive opus. By design, it is an introduction to a rapidly developing and exciting science. This text is meant as both a foundation for budding lipidologists and as a more-than-adequate, but readable, explanation of lipid biology for those practitioners who want to know more without knowing everything. We have sacrificed some scientific precision in order to more clearly make our important points, which are targeted at improving lipid management and the further prevention of premature cardiovascular disease, morbidity, and mortality.

We wrote *Lipidology, A Primer* for you to read in a few hours and to refer back to often. We tried to organize the chapters so they would conform to the way you organize your thoughts and questions. The graphic artist drew each of the schematics to be consistent with one another and fit together.

Why so few references? We were not lazy; we minimized our use of references because we want this to be a readable primer, not a definitive textbook. We have chosen instead to be as accurate as possible using widely accepted concepts, science, and results. We do include the source when we quote information from a single article or when the information or presentation is unique.

As we write this text, the 2013 ACC/AHA guideline (benefit of statin treatment depends on the dose of the statin and not the LDL achieved) is the official standard. There are several other guidelines (National Lipid Association, the European Atherosclerosis Society, the Canadian Cardiology Society) that still focus on treating to target. This difference complicates our goal of writing consistent guidance that is easy to follow. Our starting premise is a combination of both, because treating with high-dose statins often lowers LDL-C enough to reach LDL-C targets, but when that is not sufficient we believe in a reasonable attempt to reach LDL-C and non-HDL-c targets consistent with the ATP III 2004 updated recommendations. This is based on the evidence conclusively showing that "lower is indeed better."

We hope you find the book readable, and the information both concise and logically presented.

We hope this text will be the starting point of an exciting journey. We strongly encourage you to continue your lipid studies by becoming an active member of the National Lipid Association and then moving on to become Board Certified in Lipidology. But be forewarned: you cannot pass the Boards knowing only the information in this text. For that, you must take the Masters' Course of the National Lipid Association.

We share a common challenge: preventing, and hopefully stopping, the epidemic of atherosclerotic vascular disease, the leading cause of death and disability in the developed world.

We wish you pleasant reading.

Lower lipids, live longer.

— Robert Gleeson and Michael Davidson

Table of Contents

Tables

Charts

Strategies

Illustrations

A Few Important Notes

New terminology: the addition of -C and -P

Historically science and clinical research has focused on treating the total and LDL cholesterol. Increasingly, medical attention is turning to all of the potentially atherogenic apoB lipoprotein particles that contribute to the non-HDL-C. To accommodate this development, we use LDL-C and LDL-P to distinguish the LDL-Cholesterol from the LDL-Particle. If you are new to lipidology, this is new terminology, but it is an important concept.

CVD and MACE

Many terms describe the clinical results of atherosclerosis: CHD is coronary heart disease, CVD is both coronary vascular disease and cerebral vascular disease, CAD is coronary atherosclerotic disease, PAD is peripheral atherosclerotic disease, AAA is abdominal aortic aneurysms. Ouch, too confusing.

For simplicity and clarity, we use just two major abbreviations throughout this monograph. First, because coronary occlusive disease is the leading clinical presentation of a generalized vascular disease, we use CAD to abbreviate coronary atherosclerotic disease. Second, we use MACE for major adverse coronary event to include coronary, cerebral, and peripheral atherosclerotic disease and events.

These two abbreviations are not appropriate when reporting the results of major studies, because they force the results into unintended or unstudied boxes. When we report studies, we try to revert to the more accurate language used to accurately describe the study results.

Atherogenic dyslipidemia

We use the term "atherogenic dyslipidemia" to mean the triad of elevated triglycerides (and the associated cholesterol, i.e. VLDL-c), depressed HDL-C levels, and numerous small, dense LDL-P, usually with near-normal LDL-C levels but elevated non-HDL-C. This dyslipidemia triad is commonly seen in patients with either the (inherited) combined familial hyperlipidemia or the metabolic syndrome. It is clinically important because it doubles the risk of premature cardiovascular disease, and because this excess risk may remain even after the LDL-C is treated to goal with statins (the so-called "residual risk").

Normal versus optimal

Coronary vascular disease is the leading cause of death and disability in Western nations and will soon be the leading cause of death in the most of the world. This may be "normal" but it is certainly not acceptable. In this monograph, we use the word "normal" to mean the current dismal state of cardiovascular affairs—dismal because any time a preventable disease is thought of as anything close to "normal," we are all in trouble. We use the word "optimal" to describe the clinical state where risk of cardiovascular disease has been markedly reduced, or its progression halted.

Unfortunately, even using the relatively modest LDL-C and non-HDL-C goals, most high- and very high-risk patients are not adequately treated. Closing this treatment gap and treating residual risk will further lower cardiovascular risk.

Units of measurement

All measurements are in mg/dL. In some key areas, we include mmol value in parens. These will be obvious. In other instances, use the following rules to convert mg/dL to mmol/L and verse visa,

Total, LDL, and HDL cholesterol

- To convert mg/dL to mmol/L, divide the mg by 38.67 (or more quickly use 40)
- To convert mmol/L to mg/dL, multiply the mmol by 38.67

Triglycerides

- To convert mg/dL to mmol/L, divide the mg by 88.57 (or more quickly use 90)
- To convert mmol/L to mg/dL, multiply the mmol by 88.57

Table 1 Converting cholesterol and triglycerides from mg/dL to mmol/L
Note: We will discuss the optimal levels of the LDL-P and apo B lipoproteins in Chapter 4

	mg/dL	mmol/L
Total cholesterol		
Desirable	< 200	< 5.1
Borderline high	200 to 239	5.1 to 6.1
High	> 239	> 6.1
LDL cholesterol		
Optimal	< 70	< 1.8
Normal	< 100	< 2.6
Near normal	100 to 129	2.6 to 3.3
Borderline high	130 to 159	3.3 to 4.1
High	160 to 189	4.1 to 4.8
Very high	> 189	> 4.8
Non-HDL-C		
Optimal	< 100	< 2.4
Normal	< 130	< 3.2
High	190 to 219	4.8 to 5.5
Very high	> 220	> 5.5
HDL cholesterol		
Low (undesirable)	male < 40 female < 50	< 1.0 < 1.25
Normal	40 to 60	2.0 to 2.6
High (usually desirable)	> 60	> 2.6

Triglycerides		
Optimal	< 70	< 0.80
Physiologic	30 to 70	0.34 to 0.80
Normal	< 150	< 1.7
Borderline high	150 to 199	1.7 to 2.2
High	200 to 499	2.2 to 5.6
Very high	> 499	> 5.6

Statins shortened by dropping "statin"

For brevity, we will refer to all statins by their first syllables and drop the two syllables "statin" at the end of the word; e.g., atorvastatin becomes atorva.

Chapter 1
Why Treat Lipids?

THIS CHAPTER BRIEFLY SUMMARIZES the development of the lipid theory of atherosclerosis, gives a brief history of the success of lipid treatment to date, and offers an assessment of where and how far we still need to go.

Key Points

- The relationship between elevated lipids and coronary vascular disease has been established definitively. Numerous studies demonstrate that lowering LDL-C lowers events.
- Inflammation amplifies or accelerates the development of atherosclerosis. Most treatments for LDL also lower inflammation (statins, exercise, heart-healthful diet, and no smoking).
- Abnormal levels of lipids and lipoproteins cause atherosclerosis and cardiovascular disease.
- The rise in atherosclerotic disease over the past 100 years is largely the result of changes in the Western lifestyle, a lifestyle that is now spreading internationally.
- Multiple primary and secondary prevention studies have proven that lipid-lowering therapies prevent and reduce the burden of CVD.

The history of the lipid theory of atherosclerosis

The German pathologist Rudolph Virchow observed in 1856 the association between atherosclerosis and lipids. In 1904, Felix Marchand first used the term "atherosclerosis" to describe arterial obstructive disease. In 1913, the Russian Nikolai Anitzschkow (also Anichokov) demonstrated that he could induce atherosclerosis by feeding very high-cholesterol diets to rabbits.

In 1951, Duff and McMillian published an article entitled, "The Pathology of Atherosclerosis," (*Am J Med* 1951; 11: 92–108) that first used the phrase "lipid hypothesis" to describe the association between high-saturated fat diets and atherosclerotic disease. Then in 1956, Ancel Keys published "Atherosclerosis: a problem in newer public health" (*J. Mt Sinai Hospital* 1953; 20(2): 118–139). Keys hypothesized, and later showed in his *Seven Countries Study*, that a direct correlation between saturated fat consumption and serum cholesterol largely accounted for differences in the rates of atherosclerosis among countries. (Note that this correlation related to the intake of saturated fat. The total intake of fat as a percentage of daily calories has no correlation with atherosclerosis.) This saturated fat theme is suddenly an area of some dispute, so stay tuned.

Through much of the middle part of the twentieth century, atherosclerotic disease and coronary deaths were viewed as an immutable part of the aging

Table 2 Milestones from the Framingham Heart Study
http://www.framingham.com/heart/timeline.htm accessed on October 30, 2009

1948	Start of the Framingham Heart Study
1960	Cigarette smoking found to increase risk of heart disease
1961	Cholesterol and blood pressure found to increase risk of heart disease
1970	Hypertension found to increase the risk of stroke
1977	Effects of triglycerides, LDL, and HDL described
1981	Effect of diet on heart disease described
1988	High levels of HDL found to reduce risk of death
1994	Lp(a) and apo E described as possible risk factors
1997	Cumulative effects of smoking and elevated cholesterol on risk of heart disease
1998	10-year Framingham Risk Score developed

process. Of course, this was also an era when we did not know much about the risks of cigarette smoke or hypertension: in 1945, US President Franklin D. Roosevelt, who smoked cigarettes, died of malignant—and untreated—hypertension of 220/145.

The Framingham Heart Study started in 1948 to study the causes of heart disease. The Study has made major contributions to our understanding of atherosclerosis. These are summarized in the Table 2 above. Even today, Framingham Heart Study researchers continue to contribute to discovering new genes underlying major heart disease risk factors—body mass index, blood cholesterol, cigarette smoking, blood pressure and glucose/diabetes.

Even as recently as 1984, the NIH felt it necessary to hold a consensus conference to examine two basic questions: whether serum cholesterol caused atherosclerosis and whether therapeutic or large-scale dietary efforts to lower the serum cholesterol would be beneficial.

The National Cholesterol Education Program

In the 1970s, a "normal" total cholesterol was somewhere between 280 to 300, and few people had ever heard of LDL or HDL. The "acceptable" level of total cholesterol began to come down in the 1980s, moving toward 240. In the late 1980s, HDL and LDL were identified as important risk factors and moved into clinical practice. By the late 1990s, statin treatments to lower LDL-C became the focus of clinical practice and the race was on to define a level associated with plaque regression and safety. In the mid-2000s, the target LDL-C goal was linked to risk, non-HDL identified as a new treatment target, and the sole emphasis on LDL-C started to be shared with VLDL-C (the triglyceride-rich lipoprotein cholesterol within non-HDL), and LDL-P.

The 2013 ACC/AHA guidelines, based on rigid criteria for the inclusion of accepted research, determined that the benefit of treatment was based more on the dose of the statin than on the target LDL achieved. Since their publication, a major clinical trial, IMPROVE-IT validated that a non-statin (ezetimibe) lowers CAD events by the degree of LDL-C reduction, thereby supporting the "LDL hypothesis" and the mantra "lower is better." The authors concluded the results of this major trial (which contained more events than all the other major statin trials combined) should affect future guideline recommendations. The recent approval of PCSK9 inhibitors will likely spur new guidelines that return a focus to targets of therapy.

This book will focus on the practical application of all of these guidelines and developments to your clinical practice, with the goal of improving the management of your patients who are at increased risk for, or already have, atherosclerotic disease.

The causes of atherosclerosis

Atherosclerosis is not a part of normal aging. Many people with optimal cardiovascular risk profiles and health-promoting lifestyles live into old age with minimal risk of atherosclerosis. The goal of good cardiovascular prevention is to minimize risk factors to prevent the morbidity and mortality of premature atherosclerosis.

Atherosclerosis is caused by several adverse factors that promote cholesterol deposition in the arterial intima, a process that occurs slowly over many decades. Apo B lipoproteins carry cholesterol into the arterial wall; the greater the plasma concentration of apo B lipoproteins, the greater the diffusion through the endothelium and into the arterial intima. This process is affected by many non-cholesterol risk factors that increase the risk.

Many of these risk factors were identified in the INTERHEART study (Yusuf et al. *Lancet* 2004; 364: 937–952), a 52-country case-controlled study of the causes of myocardial infarcts. Interestingly and pertinent to this monograph, the INTERHEART data indicates that dyslipidemia is responsible for more than 50% of the population-attributable vascular risk.

To a p value of 0.0001, INTERHEART showed that over 90% of risk in men and 94% in women could be attributed to nine risk factors. These nine factors were associated with the risk of atherosclerotic disease in all 52 countries, in men and women, and in the young and the old. Six factors were associated with increased risk: (1) smoking, (2) raised ratio of apo B to apo A-1 (essentially the ratio of non-HDL to HDL), (3) hypertension, (4) diabetes,

(5) abdominal obesity, and (6) adverse psycho-social factors. Three factors were associated with decreased risk: (1) daily consumption of fruits and veggies, (2) regular but modest alcohol intake, and (3) regular physical activity.

Table 3 Risk Factors for Ischemic Heart Disease in > 90% of cases from INTERHEART, p > 0.0001 (Yosuf, Lancet 2004)

Risk of MI by Risk Factor	HR adjusted for age, sex, and smoking
apoB : apoA1 (Q5 to Q1)	3.87
Diabetes	3.08
Current smoking	2.95
Hypertension	2.48
Abdominal obesity	2.22
Psychosocial	2.51
Daily fruits and veggies	0.70
Daily exercise	0.72
Some alcohol	0.79

Please note that some lifestyle habits and risk factors actively promote the development of atherosclerosis, while different lifestyle habits, and risk factors actually reduce or retard the development of atherosclerosis. This distinction causes as much as a 14-year difference in life expectancy between those whose habits promote disease and those whose habits prevent disease. That's a huge difference.

Some people minimize their risk factors and maximize health-promoting activities, thus reducing their risk of future atherosclerosis. The Nurses' Health Study (Stampfer, *NEJM* 2000; 343: 16–22) followed 84,000 women for 14 years to identify the major factors that can reduce the risk of heart disease. The study identified five factors that lowered the risk of CVD by 80%. They were (1) maintaining a normal weight; (2) not using tobacco; (3) getting regular physical activity (e.g., brisk walking) for 30 minutes a day; (4) drinking at least half an alcoholic drink a day; and (5) eating a diet high in cereal fiber, marine omega-3 fats, folic acid, a high ratio of polyunsaturated to saturated fat, and low in both trans-fats and glycemic load. Unfortunately, fewer than 5% of the women followed these healthful habits.

Based on INTERHEART and the Nurses' Health Study, we can identify the markers of a disease-reducing, health-promoting person: (1) no tobacco; (2) more than 30 minutes of daily physical activity; (3) a low LDL and elevated HDL; (4) a low blood pressure; (5) no glucose intolerance; (6) maintaining a normal weight and no abdominal obesity; (7) favorable (or at least not adverse) psycho-social factors; (8) a diet with lots of fruits and veggies, omega-3 foods and oils, a high ratio of mono- and un-saturated to saturated fats, whole grains; and (9) some (but not too much) alcohol. The American Heart Association now has a "Simple 7" campaign based on these factors. We will discuss this in the lifestyle chapter of the book.

Table 4 Differentiating low- and high-risk populations

	Low risk	Increased risk
Tobacco	Never smoked	Smokes
Ratio of apo B to apo A-1	Low	High
Blood pressure	< 120/80	> 140/90 or on Rx
Blood sugar	Normal	> 100 or on Rx
Abdominal obesity	No	Present
Diet	Low ratio of saturated to un-, mono-, or poly-unsaturated fat, > 5 colorful fruits and veggies, ocean fish	High saturated and trans-fats, rare to few fruits and veggies, lots of processed foods, snacks, and soda
Physical activity	> 3.5 hours/week	Little to none
Alcohol	Some to moderate	None or excessive

The causes of atherosclerosis then fall into three big groupings. First are the medical conditions that require preventive treatments: abnormal lipids and lipoproteins, hypertension, glucose intolerance or diabetes and inflammatory disease. Second are the personal lifestyle choices that can increase or decrease the risk of heart disease: tobacco, obesity, a healthy diet, some alcohol, and physical activity. Third is a societal and governmental issue:

psycho-social factors (read poverty, illiteracy, and a lack of education), stress of living in dangerous environments. This refers to our collective responsibility to ensure that all peoples have access to health-promoting foods, and safe areas to play and exercise. Most experts agree that we must treat obesity as we did tobacco—making a societal push to reduce portion size, promote healthful eating and health-promoting foods.

As health care providers, we must focus our attention on minimizing the medical risks using treatment and promoting a healthful lifestyle. A healthful lifestyle requires both active individual participation and the support of societal and public health programs. Think of smoking, a dangerous lifestyle choice that was made socially unacceptable by public health programs, legislation, support from the American Lung and American Heart Associations, the school systems, and advertising.

The best clinical outcomes are seen in patients who both adopt a healthful lifestyle and receive preventive treatment to achieve optimal targets for all of their risk factors. The American Heart Association's Simple 7 promote these issues.

The development of atherosclerosis

Clinical atherosclerosis is the end result of a disease that develops slowly over many decades. For most of this time, atherosclerosis is a silent asymptomatic disease until it suddenly presents as a myocardial infarction or as the chronic ischemia of angina or claudication. Tragically, the sudden appearance of a plaque rupture in a coronary artery is fatal one-third of the time.

Atherosclerosis begins when risk factors become less than optimal, often in childhood. Ongoing since 1972 and in multiple publications, the Bogalusa Heart Study from Tulane University has clearly shown that the major causes of atherosclerosis start in childhood. The PDAY Study on the Natural History and Risk Factors of Atherosclerosis in Children and Youth (*Fetal and Ped Path* 2002; 21: 213–217) studied 3,000 subjects who died between age 15 and 34. This study reached three important conclusions: first, atherosclerosis begins in childhood; second, young adults often have "significant" lesions; and third, even at young ages, the risk of atherosclerosis is clearly associated with the classic cardiovascular risk factors (adverse lipid profile, tobacco, obesity and abdominal fat, diabetes, and elevated blood pressure).

These same risk factors cause atherosclerosis at all ages. But we need to ask ourselves how and why these particular risk factors cause the disease. These answers will help us better understand our treatments.

Atherosclerosis has three primary drivers: (1) elevated levels of LDL-Particles or apo B lipoprotein particles to and through an endothelium (2) which has been damaged by tobacco, hypertension, hyperglycemia, and inflammation, (3) leading macrophages within the arterial intima to perceive the oxidated (rancid) apo B lipoproteins as toxic, prompting their ingestion by macrophages, which coalesce into a foam cell, the start of an atherosclerotic lesion.

A coalescence of cholesterol-laden macrophages and foam cells is called a "fatty streak." These foam cells die, increasing the inflammatory response within the intima, which increases the migration of smooth muscle cells and more inflammation. Sometimes the fatty streak fibroses, stabilizing as a plaque that is not likely to rupture. These plaques have more collagen and less lipid, with or without calcium, and a thick fibrous cap between the fatty streaks and the endothelial side of the intima. Alternatively, other plaques are more fragile and prone to rupture. These plaques have large lipid-filled centers, with necrosis and micro-hemorrhages, moderate amounts of inflammation and enzyme activity, all covered by a thin endothelial cap that is prone to rupture.

Scientific investigators are looking at all parts of this atherosclerosis pathophysiology. But it is abundantly clear that elevated levels of LDL-C and apo B particles are primary agents that cause the disease. In fact, if serum LDL-C levels are below 50 or 60, new atherosclerotic lesions will probably not develop. There is good epidemiological and clinical data to support this theory.

We're making progress

As practitioners focused on prevention, our collective goals are to disrupt this decades-long process, to stop new or further atherosclerosis, to prevent the clinical consequences of CVD, and, someday, to reverse the disease.

The information above tells us what we must do to win this war. Success requires that we (1) treat to target abnormal lipids, lipoproteins, hypertension, elevated fasting blood sugars, and inflammation; (2) go to zero tolerance for tobacco and trans-fats, (3) minimize our societal acceptance of calorie-dense, nutritionally poor "foods"; and (4) improve our collective diets, reduce the pandemic of obesity, and increase physical activity.

We're getting there, slowly but surely.

Think back to what we have learned in just 60 years. Now think about how much has already changed: the number of people who smoke has fallen by half, the average population systolic blood pressure and serum cholesterol levels are falling. And, the mortality rate for diseases of the heart has also fallen.

The chart below shows the 50% decline in CAD 1950 to the present. This is massive.

Chart 1 Change in Age-Adjusted Death Rates 1950 to 2000

Source: NHLBI Oct. 2006

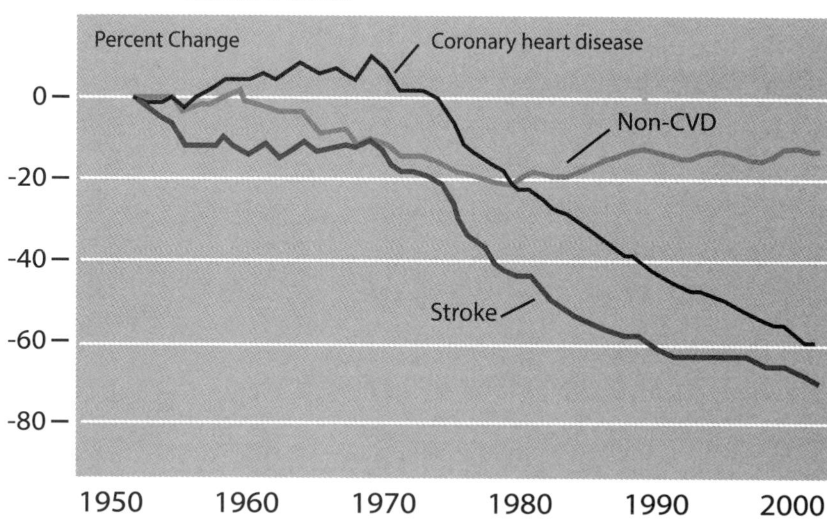

Of course, this raises the question of whether the rates of heart disease have fallen because of better intervention or better prevention. The nod goes to prevention.

Unal et al. (*Circ* 2004; 109: 1101–1107) looked at the coronary death rates in the UK from 1981 to 2000. During that time, they found that heart disease death rates fell by 62% in men and 45% in women between the ages of 25 and 84. They found that 42% of the decline occurred because of better individual treatments (heart failure treatments 13%, secondary prevention 11%, initial treatment of MI 8%, and hypertension treatment 3%); and 58% of the decline occurred because of population risk reductions (decline in smoking 48%, decline in blood pressure 9.5%, and a decline of serum cholesterol levels 9.5%). However, they noted that from 1980 to 2000, "adverse trends" were observed for physical activity, obesity, and diabetes.

Table 5 Explaining the Decrease in Deaths for Coronary Disease, 1980 to 2000 (Ford, NEJM 2007; 356: 2388–2398)

Disease treatment	
	Attributable Percentage
Initial treatment for MI or unstable angina	– 10
Revascularization and secondary prevention	– 11
Treatment of heart failure	– 9
Revascularization for angina + other	– 5
Other	– 12
Total for disease treatment	**– 47**
Primary prevention	
Reduction in total cholesterol	– 24
Reduction in systolic BP	– 20
Decreasing smoking prevalence	– 12
Increased physical activity	– 5
Total for primary prevention	**– 61**
Adverse trends	
Increasing BMI	+ 8
Increasing prevalence of diabetes	+ 10
Total for adverse trends	**+ 18**

Ford et al. (*NEJM* 2007; 356: 2388–2398) looked at the reasons for the decline in heart disease in America and compared the gains from disease treatment and primary prevention. He found similar results, giving the nod to prevention over treatment, and noting the adverse impact of the obesity and sedentary behaviors.

Prevention pays big dividends. But we face two challenges: first, as Table 4 shows, we are losing the lifestyle battle. Badly. Second, optimally treating abnormal lipids in a 60-year old who has had an MI can only slow—but not reverse—the disease that developed over a lifetime. This raises the interesting question: if you really wanted to *prevent* the development of atherosclerosis, at what age would you start to aggressively treat lipids and lower LDL-C? We do not have an answer, but the question needs to be asked. At a minimum, since atherosclerosis begins early in life, the best means to reduce CVD is likely to promote and enable heart-healthful lifestyle choices early in childhood.

The non-atherogenic state

Atherosclerosis is nearly ubiquitous in Western societies. Over the past 100 years, our diets, physical activities, and risk factors all changed dramatically. Our evolutionary genetics were not made for this Western surfeit of calories, obesity, tobacco, and a sedentary lifestyle. The current epidemic of atherosclerosis may well exist because these changes pushed our current LDL-C levels to levels twice as high as physiologically necessary in our hunter-gatherer ancestors.

Our biological enzyme processes of lipoprotein metabolism originated in our hunter-gatherer forbearers, who, during alternating periods of feast and famine, had to conserve energy and maintain minimum cholesterol and triglyceride levels. Today's metabolic problems, including atherosclerosis, stem from our current state of a near constant excess of calories, fat, and lack of activity.

Studies of primitive cultures or hunter-gatherers show that low-risk populations can and do exist. At one point in time, and not very long ago, all of our ancestors were hunter-gatherers. Studies of modern primitive hunter-gatherer cultures show low, and probably physiologic, lipid levels.

Some genetically blessed people simply do not develop atherosclerosis. They have inherited a heterozygous hypobetalipoproteinemia; their LDL-C ranges from 25 to 40, and they have no biologic or developmental problems. Other lucky souls inherit loss of function mutations in PCSK9 or the NPC1L1 enzyme and have a lifetime of lowered LDL and significantly lower rates of atherosclerosis.

Table 6 Lipid levels in primitive cultures and others
Adapted from O'Keefe JACC; 2142–2146 (2004)

	Total cholesterol	LDL-C
People heterozygous for hypobetalipoproteinemia (apo B)	80	30 to 50
Newborn		30 to 70
Hazda	110	
Inuit	145	
Pygmy	105	
American adult	208	130

As we focus on preventing or treating atherosclerosis, we need to address the key problem that complicates and hinders the effectiveness of our medications: our modern lifestyle promotes atherosclerosis. We eat a diet of calorie-dense, refined, and processed foods high in saturated and trans-fats and salt, but low in nutritional value. We are sedentary, inactive, and obese. We have rampant levels of insulin resistance and diabetes. Twenty percent of the population still smokes; and half of all hypertensives are not adequately treated.

But not all is lost in the fight to control atherosclerosis. Success in this battle is being driven by advances in the science of both lipidology and vascular biology, and the multiplicity of effective medical treatments of lipids. Someday we might, just might, be able to look back and wonder why we tolerated such high levels of atherosclerotic mortality and morbidity for so long. Asking that question is the subject of this book.

Section I

Lipid and Atherosclerosis Essential Biology

Chapter 2

Lipoprotein Biochemistry

This chapter is a first—but important—step to better understanding serum lipids, lipoproteins, and their biochemical pathways. These concepts will set the stage for later chapters, which discuss how lipoproteins lead to disease and how to best treat each lipid disorder.

You need to understand lipoprotein biology, because the commonly measured serum cholesterol and triglycerides are carried in these lipoproteins, abnormalities of the lipoprotein-related enzymes lead to disease, and lipid-modifying treatments are focused on these key enzymes. And, most importantly, the apo B lipoproteins carry cholesterol through the arterial endothelium and into the intima to cause atherosclerosis.

Key Points

- Cholesterol and triglyceride are hydrophobic fats that must be packaged (emulsified) in hydrophilic lipoproteins for transport in plasma.
- The amount of cholesterol and triglyceride carried by each of the lipoproteins varies by lifestyle choices, inherited lipid disease, other diseases, and medications.
- Lipoprotein particles are identified by their surface apo-lipoproteins, which also serve as ligands to activate or inhibit enzymes.

- All lipoprotein particles that carry an apo B (VLDL, IDL, LDL, and Lp(a)) are atherogenic. Particles with apo A-I or A-II (HDL) on their surface are usually (but not always) anti-atherogenic.
- Lipoprotein particles either are related to each other or interact with each other.
- Lipoprotein particles are increasingly important in the thorough diagnosis and treatment of lipid disorders.

NOTE: Unless otherwise noted, all comments below refer to the status of lipoproteins in a non-pathologic state.

Good lipid management requires an understanding of both (1) cholesterol and triglyceride, and (2) all of the lipoproteins that ferry these lipids around the body. To better understand how lipoproteins lead to disease and how to best treat each lipid disorder, we must first understand the lipoproteins that carry cholesteryl ester and triglyceride.

Labs measure, and we usually treat, the serum level of cholesterol or triglycerides. This is appropriate because, under physiologic conditions, the lipoprotein LDL-Particles carry 90% of the cholesterol and the lipoprotein VLDL-Particles carry 90% of the triglyceride.

At the get-go and to really shake up your thinking about cholesterol, consider that lipidology should probably be the concern of gastroenterologists. The gut produces both nascent apo A-1 (used to make HDL) and chylomicrons that carry triglyceride and cholesteryl ester from the jejunum to the cells and liver. The liver controls plasma levels of lipids by modulating the metabolism of VLDL-P; the catabolism of IDL-P, LDL-P, and HDL-P; and the formation of cholesterol-laden bile acids, which are secreted back into the gut.

The liver is intimately involved in almost every step of lipid metabolism:

1. The liver converts FFAs to triglycerides (the driver of lipoprotein production) and adds cholesterol to make VLDL-P, which is secreted into the blood circulation, acted upon by lipoprotein lipases to

remove free fatty acids, and can be viewed as the grandfather of the LDL-P.

2. The number of LDL-Receptors (LDL-R) on the surface of the liver determines the plasma level of LDL-C. The enzyme PCSK9 determines the number of LDL-R.
3. The liver surface SRB-1 receptor offloads cholesterol from HDL-P as part of reverse cholesterol transport.
4. And the liver metabolizes the cholesterol returned from both LDL-P and HDL-P into bile for secretion into the gut.

Let's read on to see how lipoprotein particles are interrelated and control the serum levels of lipids.

Lipoprotein basics

All lipoproteins have a core of hydro*phobic* cholesteryl ester and triglycerides surrounded by a hydro*philic* surface coat of phospholipids and apo-lipoproteins. Some of the surface apo-lipoproteins identify the different types of lipoprotein while others provide enzymatic ligands to facilitate the process of biochemical lipid balance and cellular function.

Each of the lipoprotein types has many functions: carrying various amounts of cholesterol and triglyceride; interacting with the endothelium; and interacting with each other to maintain cellular homeostasis—maintaining it, that is, until our Western lifestyle, genetic disorders, other diseases, or medications cause things to go terribly awry.

See illustration 1 for a drawing of the basic lipoprotein structure, which we have simplified considerably; in reality, each lipoprotein has a multitude of identifying and enzyme-activating surface apo-lipoproteins.

Let's start by looking at the individual lipoproteins and then we'll look at how they interact with each other. The names of the lipoproteins and apo-lipoproteins will become important later as we start to classify diseases and identify treatments targeted to a specific part of the process. On page 168, you will find a table listing all of the important enzymes, lipoproteins, and apo-lipoproteins mentioned in the book.

Illustration 1 Basic structure of all lipoproteins

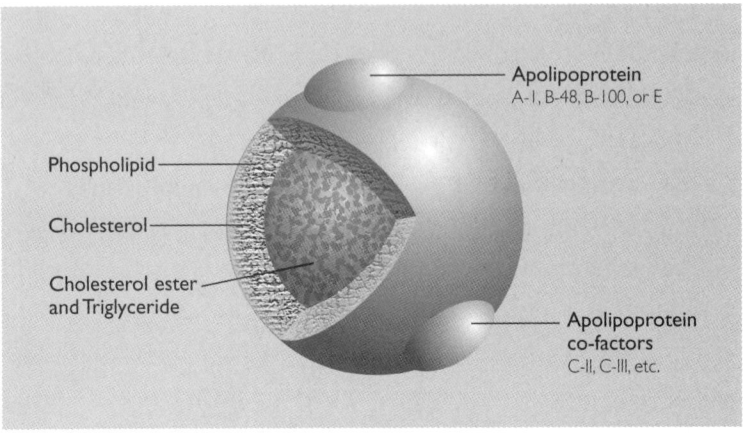

Lipoproteins can be split into two groups:

1. The atherogenic lipoproteins: these all have either an apo B-48 (chylomicrons or chylomicron remnants) or an apo B-100 (VLDL-P, IDL-P, LDL-P, and Lp(a)).
2. The anti-atherogenic lipoproteins (HDL): these all contain apo A-1 or apo A-2.

Genetics, other medical conditions, medications, and lifestyle influence both the number and content of the lipoproteins, which, in turn, cause or prevent CVD.

Illustration 2 The different classes of lipoproteins

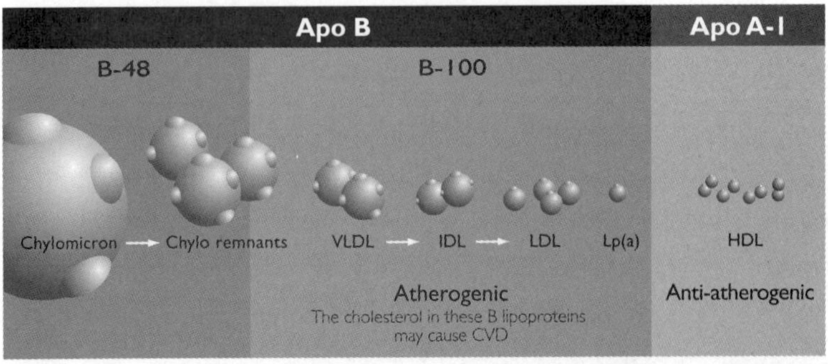

Each lipoprotein is characterized by specific surface apo-lipoproteins. These are listed in the Table 6 below. You should remember that apo B-48 is a chylomicron; apoB-100 or apoB is all of VLDL-P, IDL-P, LDL-P, or Lp(a), and apo A-1 is HDL-P.

Table 7 Lipoproteins and their major surface apo-lipoproteins

Lipoprotein	Major surface apo-lipoproteins
Chylomicron	B-48, E, C-I, C-II, A-I, A-II
Chylomicron remnants	B-48, E
VLDL	B-100, E, C-1, C-II
IDL	B-100, E
LDL	B-100
Lp(a)	B-100, (a)
HDL	A-I, A-II, A-IV, C-I, C-II, D, E

The atherogenic lipoproteins

All of the atherogenic lipoproteins contain one apo B per lipoprotein: intestinally-produced apo B-48 on chylomicrons and chylomicron remnants; and hepatic-produced apo B-100 on VLDL, IDL, LDL, and Lp(a). We typically focus on the cholesterol in LDL-P (the LDL-C), but the cholesterol in all of the apo B lipoproteins—including the chylomicron remnants, VLDL, IDL (VLDL remnants), and LDL—can be atherogenic. We call the potentially atherogenic cholesterol in all of the apoB lipoproteins non-HDL. More later on this.

The chylomicron and chylomicron remnants

- A chylomicron carries hydrophobic triglycerides and cholesterol from the gut into the lymphatics. The chylomicron, surrounded by a single layer of hydrophilic phospholipid cholesterol and several key apo-lipoproteins, moves into the lymphatics and then the systemic circulation to deliver fatty acids to muscle or fat cells. The remaining chylomicron remnants are taken up by the liver.

- When first produced, a chylomicron is 90% triglyceride and 10% cholesterol.
- Under normal conditions, the triglyceride in a chylomicron is metabolized and the chylomicron catabolized within 30 minutes of finishing a meal.

Chylomicron formation

The chylomicron is a large lipoprotein made in the wall of the jejunum. Chylomicrons ferry triglycerides and cholesterol from the gut. They deliver triglycerides for energy or fat storage to the peripheral adipose and muscle tissues, and then, as a much smaller remnant, they deliver their cholesterol to the liver. Under normal physiologic conditions, the chylomicron has a short half-life of 30 minutes before the triglycerides have been hydrolyzed away and the chylomicron remnant is taken up by the B/E receptors on the surface of the liver.

After a meal, the chylomicron is 90% triglyceride and 10% cholesterol. The outer wall of the chylomicron contains its identifying and gut-produced apo-lipoprotein apo B-48; apo E; the ligands apo C-II and apo C-III, which control the rate of hydrolysis; and apo A-I and A-II, which break away and later form HDL-P. After most of the triglyceride is hydrolyzed, the apo E on the chylomicron remnant efficiently attaches to the E part of the B/E or LDL-Receptor on the surface of the liver where the chylomicron remnant is catabolized.

The hepatic LDL-Receptor is also called the LDL-R or LDL-B/E receptor because it attaches to both apo B and apo E. By tradition, lipidologists refer to this receptor as the LDL-R. In descending order of preference, the LDL-R attaches to apo E3 and apo E4; then, and with less efficiently, to apo B; and then poorly to apo E2/E2.

LDL-R is the key player in the control of serum cholesterol and lipoprotein particle levels because the number of LDL-R determines the rate at which LDL-C and LDL-P are removed from systemic circulation. LDL-R attaches to and delipidates cholesterol from chylomicrons, chylomicron remnants, VLDL-P, IDL-P, and LDL-P.

Chylomicron catabolism

Hydrolysis of triglyceride from the chylomicron requires lipoprotein lipase LPL, which is located on the endothelial lining of cardiac and skeletal muscles and adipose tissue. The hydrolysis process is controlled by the ligands apoC-II and apoC-III. ApoC-II activates and apoC-III de-activates hydrolysis by LPL. This turn-on-and-off process is necessary to ensure that triglyceride is delivered to all parts of the body as the chylomicron tumbles through the circulation. As the chylomicron loses triglyceride, it decreases to perhaps 10% of its original volume, becoming a chylomicron remnant. As the chylomicron loses volume and surface area, apo A-I, apo A-II, and apo A-IV, break free to contribute to nascent HDL.

Abnormalities of chylomicron metabolism

When chylomicrons are not efficiently and quickly removed from plasma, the triglyceride level rises to pathological levels. The two primary abnormalities of chylomicron metabolism that cause hypertriglyceridemia include (1) genetically deficient or absent LPL or (2) deficient or absent LPL activating factor apo C-II.

In most patients with hyperchylomicronemia, the plasma triglyceride levels exceed 1,000, saturating the LPL, and exacerbating the hypertriglyceridemia. The serum from these patients forms a creamy layer after spending the night in the lab refrigerator.

VLDL and IDL (intermediate density lipoprotein or VLDL remnants)

- VLDL-P carries triglyceride, cholesterol, and key apo-proteins from the liver.
- Leaving the liver, VLDL is normally 60% triglyceride and 12% cholesterol, making a 5:1 ratio. The remaining 28% is protein and phospholipid.
- The hydrolysis of triglyceride from the VLDL makes the VLDL a smaller lipoprotein, which we call a VLDL remnant or intermediate density lipoprotein (IDL). These remnant VLDL lipoproteins are very atherogenic.

- Half of IDL-P is taken up by the LDL-R. The other half is further hydrolyzed by hepatic lipase (HL), so that the only remaining surface apo-lipoprotein is apo B. We know this particle as LDL-P.

VLDL-P metabolism

VLDL-P is produced in the liver by the combination of apoB-100 proteins, which the liver produces in abundance, and free fatty acids (FFA), which are formed into triglycerides by the enzyme DGAT or diglyceride acyl transferase. The enzyme microsomal transfer protein (MTP) is essential to package the triglycerides, cholesterol, and apoB together. VLDL-P ferries triglycerides to the systemic tissues for energy or storage. Under physiologic conditions, 60% of each VLDL-P is triglyceride, the remainder is cholesterol.

When exiting the liver, each VLDL-P carries a large amount of triglyceride and a small amount of cholesterol surrounded by an outer wall of phospholipids, apoB-100, apoC-I, apoC-II, apoC-III, and apoE.

Hydrolysis of the triglyceride in the VLDL-P

The triglyceride in the VLDL-P is initially hydrolyzed by lipoprotein lipase, LPL, the same enzyme that hydrolyzes the triglyceride from chylomicrons into free fatty acids. As with chylomicrons, apo C-II activates and C-III inhibits LPL, ensuring that the VLDL tumbles through the blood stream to all parts of the body. As the VLDL is hydrolyzed, it shrinks and sheds some of its apo-lipoproteins. This intermediate size VLDL is a VLDL remnant or IDL.

This IDL can follow either of two pathways. It can be taken up by the hepatic LDL-R *or* further hydrolyzed by hepatic lipase HL. If the IDL is further hydrolyzed, it loses all surface apo-lipoproteins except apo B and becomes an LDL—the only lipoprotein with only a single apo on its surface: apoB. In general, half of all IDL is taken up by the liver LDL-R and half becomes an LDL-particle. VLDL has a half-life of a few hours before it is hydrolyzed to an LDL-P or taken up by the hepatic LDL-R.

Illustration 3 Formation of VLDL-P, IDL-P, and LDL-P

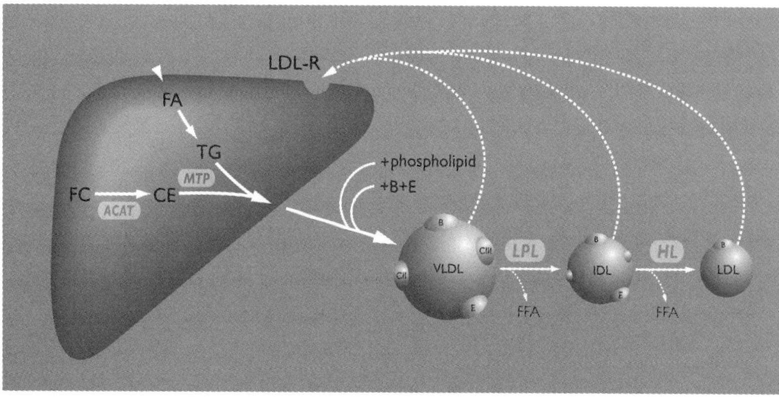

FC = free cholesterol, CE = cholesteryl ester, FA = fatty acid, TG = triglyceride, B + E = the apoB and apoE, LPL = lipoprotein lipase, HL = hepatic lipase

Abnormalities of VLDL

VLDLs, as the primary systemic carrier vehicle of triglycerides, can cause hypertriglyceridemia two ways: either (1) when they are produced in excess or (2) when not efficiently removed from the plasma. VLDL production increases in the metabolic syndrome or when we consume dietary excess of fats and refined sugars, increasing production of free fatty acids (FFAs).

As with chylomicrons, the efficient removal of VLDL is hampered whenever (1) plasma triglycerides exceed 500 mg saturating the LPL, (2) when the LPL is genetically deficient or absent, or (3) when the LPL activating factor apo C-II is deficient or absent. The serum from these patients is opalescent, in contrast to the creamy layer seen with chylomicronemia.

Elevated levels of triglyceride complicate the metabolic lipid biology and physiologic pathways by promoting an exchange of triglyceride in VLDL-P for cholesterol in IDL-P, LDL-P and HDL-P. This process leads both to small, dense LDL-P, which are now too small to be recognized and removed by LDL-R; and to small HDL-P, which shed an apo A-1, which, in turn, is excreted in the urine. This one-for-one exchange is handled by an enzyme called CETP or cholesteryl ester transfer protein.

Illustration 4 CETP exchanges triglyceride from TG-rich VLDL-P for cholesteryl ester in HDL-P and IDL-P and LDL-P

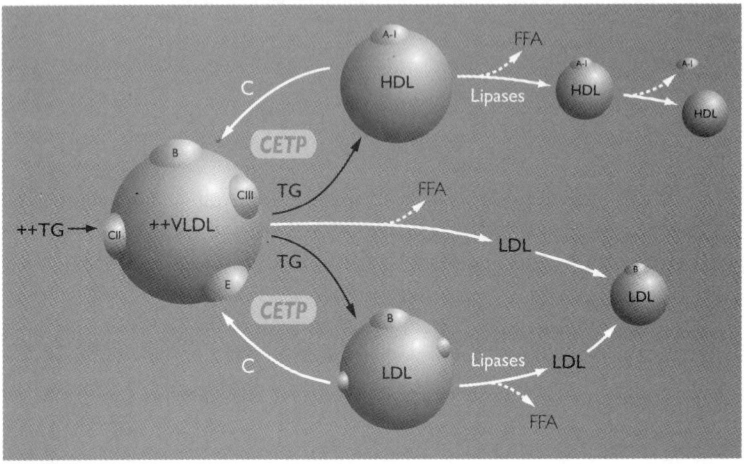

We will explore further the clinical implications of this exchange in the chapter on cardiometabolic risk.

Low Density Lipoprotein particles LDL-P

- LDL-P is an LDL particle and LDL-C is the cholesterol carried in LDL-P. They are not the same and in some diseases may be very discordant.
- Typically ninety percent of the atherogenic apo B particles are LDL-P. (The other atherogenic lipoproteins are VLDL, VLDL remnants and Lp(a).)
- LDL-P under physiologic conditions contains 90% cholesterol and 10% triglyceride. This explains why LDL-C was a good marker for atherosclerosis—but why in an era of obesity and insulin resistance, LDL-C is less predictive.
- In some patients with metabolic syndrome, the LDL-P may only carry 60% cholesterol, the rest having been replaced by triglyceride through the action of CETP.
- The only surface apo-lipoprotein on LDL is apoB, an apo-lipoprotein that is least favored by the hepatic LDL-R (LDL-Receptor). This

means that LDL-P is not efficiently removed from the circulation and circulates for two or three days.

- LDL-P stays in circulation longer than other apoB particles, and has the highest concentration of cholesterol ester making it a key cause of atherosclerosis.

LDL metabolism

As discussed above LDL-P is the grandchild of VLDL-P, formed after LPL and HL have hydrolyzed the triglycerides out of the VLDL-P and IDL-P. Under normal physiologic conditions (read, no insulin resistance or excess triglycerides), the LDL-P carries 90% of the circulating cholesterol ester. We traditionally have called this LDL-Cholesterol. This relationship falls apart in patients with insulin resistance or excess triglycerides, where LDL-P may be filled with 60% cholesterol ester and 40% triglycerides.

LDL-P pathways and pathology

The primary physiologic function of LDL-P is to distribute cholesterol for cellular membrane synthesis or for the synthesis of steroid hormones.

Each LDL-P has two possible endings. First, the apo B on the LDL can attach to the LDL-R on the liver where it is catabolized, the cholesterol ester remade either into cholesterol for another run through the VLDL pathway *or* into bile acids. Second, LDL-P can adhere to and diffuse through the endothelium into the vascular intima where the cholesterol will be oxidized to start the process that we call atherosclerosis. See illustration 6 on page 29 below and follow the two LDL-P pathways.

Lp(a)

Lp(a) is a complex and little understood lipoprotein. It is a modified apo B (LDL-P like) with an apo-lipoprotein (a) attached. The level of Lp(a) is inherited. Elevated levels of Lp(a) are atherogenic and may be associated with premature disease.

Lp(a) is genetically different from all other lipoproteins. First, Lp(a) represents a link between the atherogenicity of LDL-C and the thrombotic tendencies of plasminogen. Lp(a) has genetic components of both LDL-P and an apo(a) genetically similar to plasminogen. This places Lp(a) at the intersection of much of the pathology of atherosclerosis. Second, the level of Lp(a) is genetically determined. Neither environmental factors nor pharmacology appears to impact the levels of Lp(a). Third, we do not yet understand the metabolism or the catabolism of Lp(a), or its real relationship to atherosclerosis. But stay tuned, there is more to learn.

LDL-R metabolism

The LDL-Receptor removes apoB particles from systemic circulation. The LDL-R sits in clathrin-coated pits on the hepatic cell surface. When bound to an apoB particle, the clathrin-coated vesicle is internalized and the cholesterol removed by endocytosis. Once the cholesterol is removed, the receptor is either recycled back to the surface or destroyed. The synthesis of new LDL-R is regulated by the level of free intracellular cholesterol.

Illustration 5 LDL-R recycles to remove LDL-P from circulation (left side) until PCSK9 attaches to the LDL-R causing its catabolism (right side)

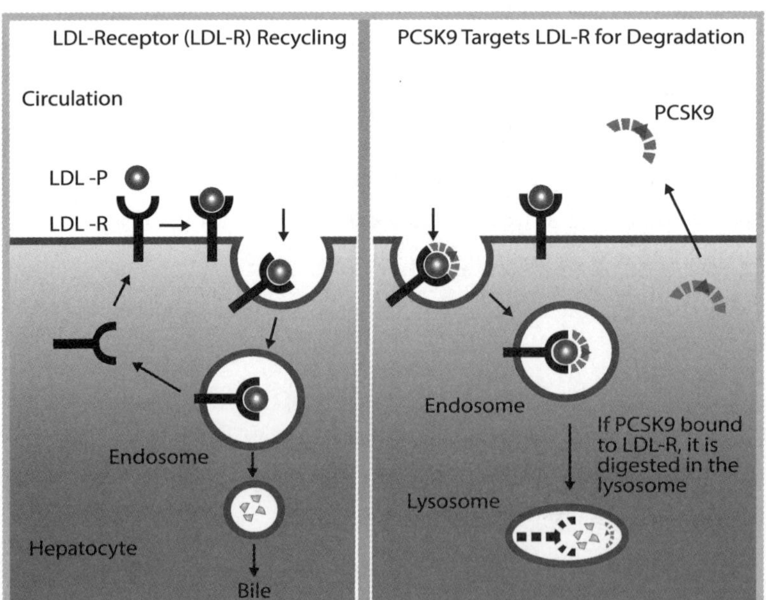

The catabolism of LDL-R is controlled by an enzyme PCSK9. When PCSK9 binds to an LDL-R, the shape of the internalized LDL-R is changed and it cannot return to cell surface and is therefore destroyed in a lysozyme.

This is shown in illustration 5 above. On the left-hand side, the LDL-R is grabbing an LDL-P from the circulation and bringing it into and the hepatocyte where the cholesterol is made into bile or recycled back to a VLDL-P. The LDL-R recycles back to the surface to repeat the process. On the right-hand side, when PCSK9 attaches to the LDL-R, it removes its last LDL-P from circulation and is then catabolized.

Increased levels of PCSK9 reduce the number of functioning LDL-R and increase the body's cholesterol level. PCSK9 levels are increased by gain of function mutations, and counterintuitively, both statins and fibrates. Decreased levels of PCSK9 reduce the catabolism of LDL-R, so there are more LDL-R on the surface to reduce the serum cholesterol level. PCSK9 levels can be decreased by loss of function mutations or blocked by the new PCSK9 inhibitor medications.

Non-atherogenic lipoproteins

The term "non-atherogenic lipoprotein" really means HDL-P, a highly complex lipoprotein with multiple functions, some of which are just now being elucidated. HDL-P carries HDL-C from arterial wall macrophages back to the liver. HDL-P may have one to four surface apo A-1(s) or apo A-2(s) per particle.

A word of caution: HDL-C is not always anti-atherogenic. There are many patients with very high levels of HDL-C who have atherosclerosis and where the elevated HDL-C was not protective. How and what is happening in these cases is not yet understood. There are no commercially available tests to measure HDL function.

High Density Lipoprotein HDL

- HDL-P is the HDL particle and HDL-C is the cholesterol carried within the HDL-P.
- The primary function of HDL-P is to ferry cholesterol ester to the steroidogenic organs.

- HDL-P far outnumber all other lipoproteins, but each HDL-P is small and carries only a small amount of cholesterol.

HDL Metabolism

HDL is a complex lipoprotein that is usually—but, as we said, not always—anti-atherogenic. The primary biologic functions of HDL-P are to (1) deliver cholesterol ester to the steroidogenic organs (adrenal, testes, and ovaries) and (2) carry cholesterol from the arterial intima back to the liver for reprocessing into bile or back into a VLDL-P for another run through systemic circulation. This process is called the reverse cholesterol transport.

HDL has many anti-atherogenic functions

HDL-P (1) is responsible for reverse cholesterol transport from a cholesterol-laden macrophage in the intima back to the liver; (2) promotes vascular dilatation; (3) preserves a well-functioning endothelium by increasing nitric oxide production; is both (4) an anti-oxidant and (5) anti-inflammatory; and inhibits (6) thrombosis, (7) endothelial cell adhesion, and both (8) vascular and (9) cellular adhesion molecules.

HDL is responsible for reverse cholesterol transport

The most important anti-atherogenic function of HDL is reverse cholesterol transport (RCT). HDL starts as a nascent non-lipidated apo A-1 molecule. This molecule maybe (1) produced in the jejunum or liver, (2) formed as a break-away by-product of chylomicron hydrolysis, or (3) released and recirculated after hepatic delipidation of a mature HDL-P.

This nascent apo A-1 comes in contact through the endothelium with a cholesterol-laden macrophage, which activates an ABCA-1 enzyme. The ABCA-1 releases free cholesterol from the macrophage to the nascent A-1. As the cholesterol joins the apo A-1, the LCAT enzyme esterifies the cholesterol, moving the hydrophobic fat into the center of the now-maturing HDL, which then gathers surface phospholipid to make a hydrophilic surface coat. Other intimal macrophage enzymes such as ABCA-4 directly contribute cholesterol ester to the enlarging HDL-P.

The HDL-P, which is now laden with cholesterol from the vessel intima, then returns the cholesterol ester to the SR-B1 receptor on the surface of the liver. Here the HDL-P is delipidated and the apo A-1 re-enters the circulation to repeat the process.

Illustration 6 Formation of HDL-P and the reverse cholesterol transport process

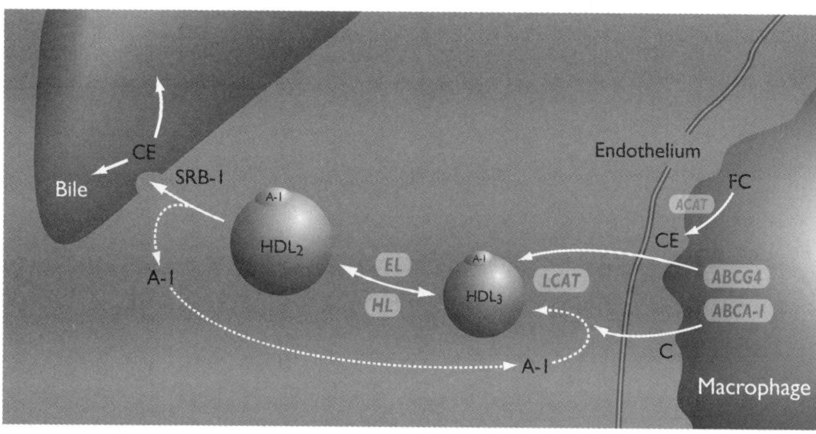

The mature HDL-P can rid itself of cholesterol in one of two ways. First, the mature HDL-P can directly carry its cholesterol ester to either the SR-B1 receptor on either (1) the liver or (2) steroidogenic tissues (adrenals, ovaries, or testes). The SR-B1 receptor delipidates the cholesterol ester from HDL-P, freeing the apo A-1 back into circulation, where the cycle is repeated. Or the enzyme CETP (cholesterol ester transfer protein) exchanges the cholesterol ester in HDL-P for triglycerides in the VLDL-P. The cholesterol ester that moved from HDL-P to LDL-P where it again has two possible outcomes: first, it may be ferried back to the hepatic LDL-R and be removed, or second, it can be carried back to the endothelium to cause more havoc.

Illustration 7 The interplay between circulating lipoproteins, the liver, and the endothelium

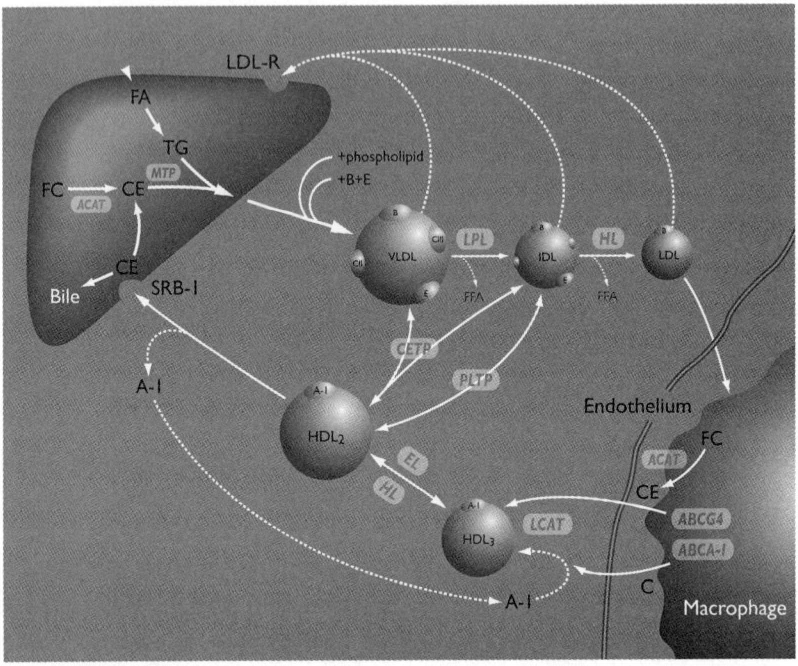

Chapter 3

Vascular Biology and Atherosclerosis

UNDERSTANDING THE VASCULAR BIOLOGY that leads to atherosclerosis offers several new potential therapeutic targets: opportunities to stabilize the endothelium and vulnerable plaques, and reduce inflammation and thrombosis.

- The cholesterol in the apoB (non-HDL) lipoproteins causes atherosclerosis by infiltrating the vascular intima.
- Atherosclerosis develops silently over decades, but often presents as a catastrophic acute thrombotic event.
- The main drivers of atherosclerosis are (1) increased numbers of apoB particles, (2) a loss of endothelial integrity, and (3) a heightened inflammatory response within the lesion.

As we noted earlier, atherosclerosis is a common disease in the developed world because our diet and sedentary lifestyle promote hypertension, insulin resistance, and serum lipid levels far above physiological requirement.

The rate of atherosclerotic development is neither linear nor predictable. Some early fatty streaks and plaques resolve while others progress. At any time, an arterial vascular tree may have lesions running the entire spectrum from fatty streaks to lipid-laden, thin-capped, rupture-prone plaques, to calcified inactive plaques.

The process that leads to atherosclerosis is a natural biologic response to high levels of sterols, including cholesterol, which the body perceives as toxic when in the arterial wall. Excess levels of cholesterol are removed from most interstitial tissues by the lymphatics—with the exception of the arterial intima, the only tissue that lacks lymphatic drainage. In all other parts of the body, lymphatics remove cholesterol so effectively that non-vascular tissue levels of cholesterol are often only 10% of the serum level.

When apo B containing lipoproteins break through the endothelium into the arterial intima, they bind to proteoglycans, become oxidized, and are taken up by monocytes or macrophages to form foam cells. This inflammatory response begins as the intima tries to protect itself from what it perceives as a toxic chemical: cholesterol.

A healthy endothelium, a smooth sheet-like, one-cell thick membrane measuring 0.001 mm, promotes vascular health. It is the only tissue in the body that does not promote coagulation or cellular adhesion. A healthy endothelium produces nitric oxide to dilate arteries and reduces inflammation and oxidation.

Table 8 Endothelium, healthy or diseased

	Healthy endothelium	Diseased endothelium
Diameter	Dilated	Constricted
Growth	Inhibited	Promoted
Thrombosis	Anti	Pro
Inflammatory	Anti	Pro
Oxidant	Anti	Pro

The endothelium is easily damaged by the all-too-common risk factors including hypercholesterolemia, hypertension, diabetes, and smoking. A diseased endothelium is dysfunctional and exacerbates the development of atherosclerosis. Once the endothelium is damaged, a process starts that is akin to "the old man who swallowed the shoe."

A damaged endothelium and intima produces less nitric oxide (constricting arteries and making them less pliable), is more permeable to monocytes and apo B particles, expresses more adhesion molecules, is pro-thrombotic, and promotes the activity of adhesion molecules (e.g., VCAM) and the inflammatory Lp-PLA-2.

Illustration 8 Development of an early atherosclerotic lesion

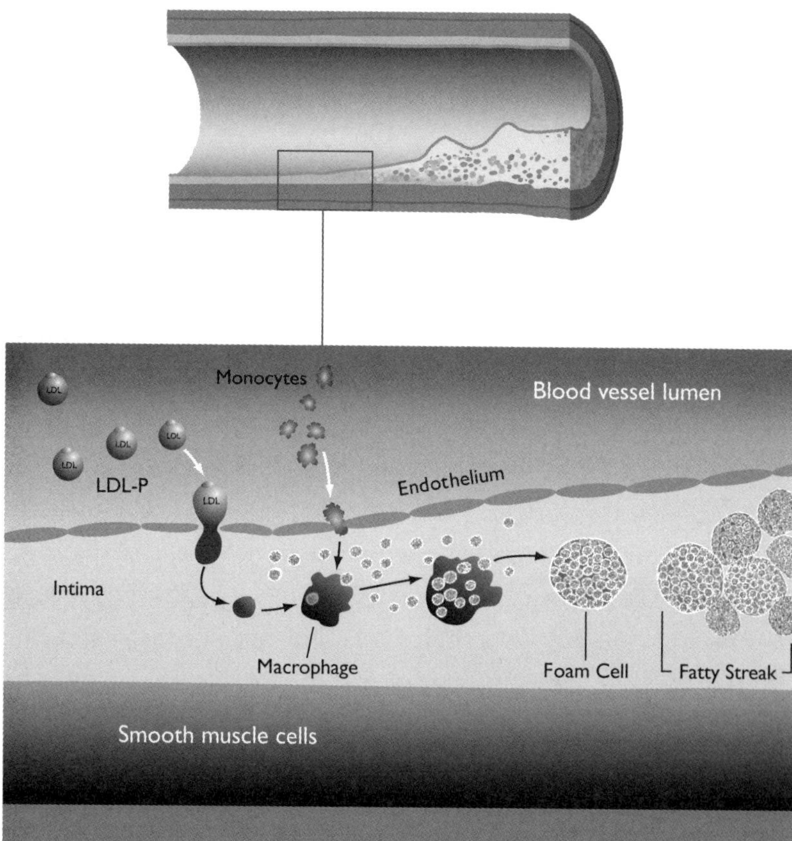

The damaged endothelium releases adhesion molecules that encourage monocytes and LDL-particles to enter the subendothelial space. Once there, the LDL-particles and cholesterol esters are oxidized, making them more inflammatory and causing more macrophage reaction. The monocytes differentiate into macrophages and engulf the toxic cholesterol, forming foam cells, which then coalesce into fatty streaks.

In turn, the activated, cholesterol-rich macrophages release (think of this as a call for more help) chemicals including chemo-attractants and cytokines (tumor-necrosing factor α and interleukins). These oxidized sterols are toxic to cells and activate nuclear regulatory factors which turn on ABCA-1/ABCG-1 to efflux cholesterol from the cells onto nascent apo A-I, the start of reverse cholesterol transport.

The macrophages also recruit smooth muscle cells from the lamina propria, which secrete extracellular matrix components in an attempt to stabilize the lesion. This is countered by the macrophages, which secrete metalloproteinases that degrade the extracellular matrix, which results in arterial wall remodeling leading to stenosis or aneurysmal formation. Metalloproteinases are also thought to weaken the "cap" covering an atherosclerotic lesion leading to rupture and an acute event.

Other enzymes seek to balance this inflammatory activity. This balance between plaque stabilization and dissolution becomes a key focus in promoting or preventing an acute event, because once a plaque ruptures, an intravascular thrombus forms.

Some plaques are fibrotic, calcified, and unlikely to rupture, while others with thin caps are unstable and prone to rupture. A stable plaque is fibrotic, may be calcified, has a small lipid core, a poor vascular supply, little to no macrophage activity, and neither Lp-PLA2 nor metalloproteinase activity. An unstable or vulnerable plaque that is prone to rupture has a thin cap, an enlarging lipid-macrophage core, substantial metalloproteinase activity (chewing away at the cap), active macrophages, a paucity of smooth muscle cells and, often, internal neovascularization with hemorrhage into the plaque. An increased serum level of Lp-PLA2 indicates active inflammation in metabolically active or vulnerable plaques.

Illustration 9 An unstable and a stable plaque

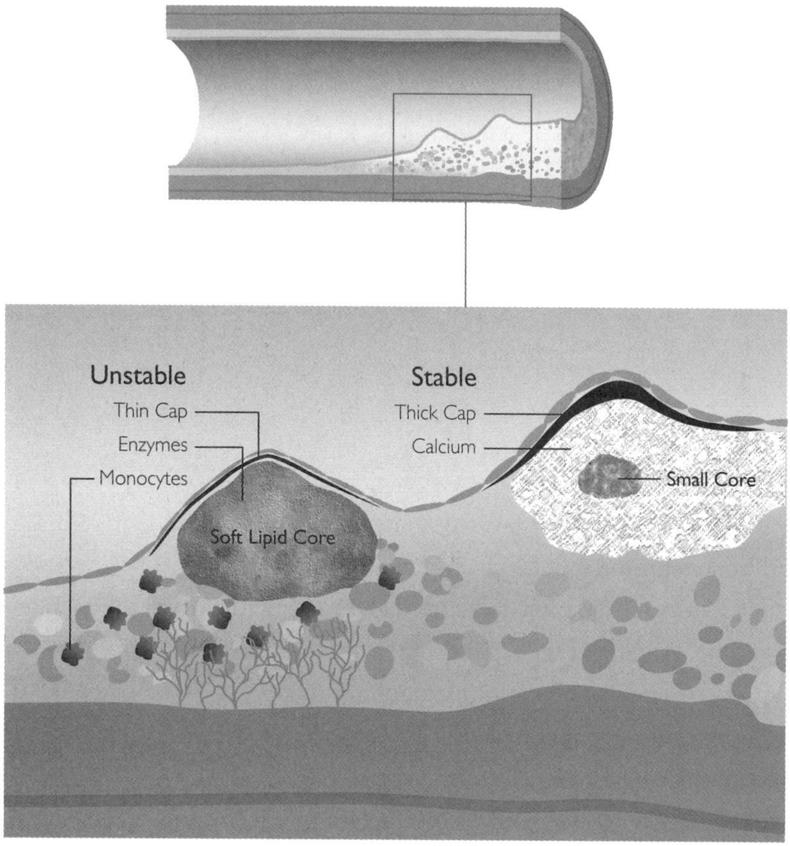

The size of the plaque has almost nothing to do with whether it ruptures. Fully two-thirds of acute coronary events arise from non-critical plaques (often called luminal irregularities) that only cause 20% to 40% luminal occlusion. Upon rupture, a plaque releases potent pro-coagulants and inflammatory cells that cause rapid propagation of an intra-luminal clot. If the thrombus only partially occludes the lumen, the patient experiences unstable angina or a non-ST-segment-elevating myocardial infarction (NSTEMI). Alternatively, a clot that completely occludes the lumen produces an ST-segment-elevating MI (STEMI).

Illustration 10 A vulnerable plaque ruptures spewing its contents into the arterial lumen and starting the clotting cascade

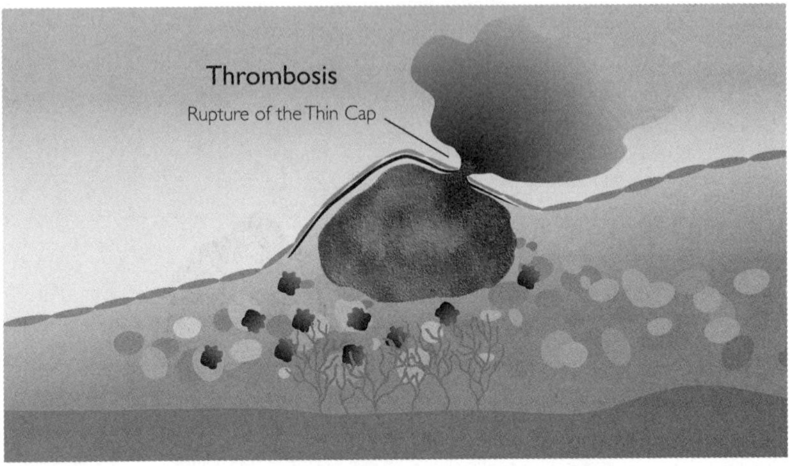

Plaque rupture becomes the business of the emergency medical technician, the emergency room physician, and the invasive cardiologist. Or, as happens all too often, a plaque rupture becomes the business of the undertaker.

Preventing the plaque development and rupture is the business of all clinicians who see patients at risk for atherosclerosis—and right now that basically means everyone.

The goals of good lipid management are to (1) stop new plaque development, (2) stop the growth of existing of plaques, (3) reduce the inflammatory processes in the plaques, (4) stabilize existing atherosclerotic lesions, and (5) prevent cardiovascular events and premature morbidity and mortality.

Illustration 11 The goals of lipid treatment are to stop new plaque development or growth and to stabilize existing lesions (adapted from DeGomaMD.com)

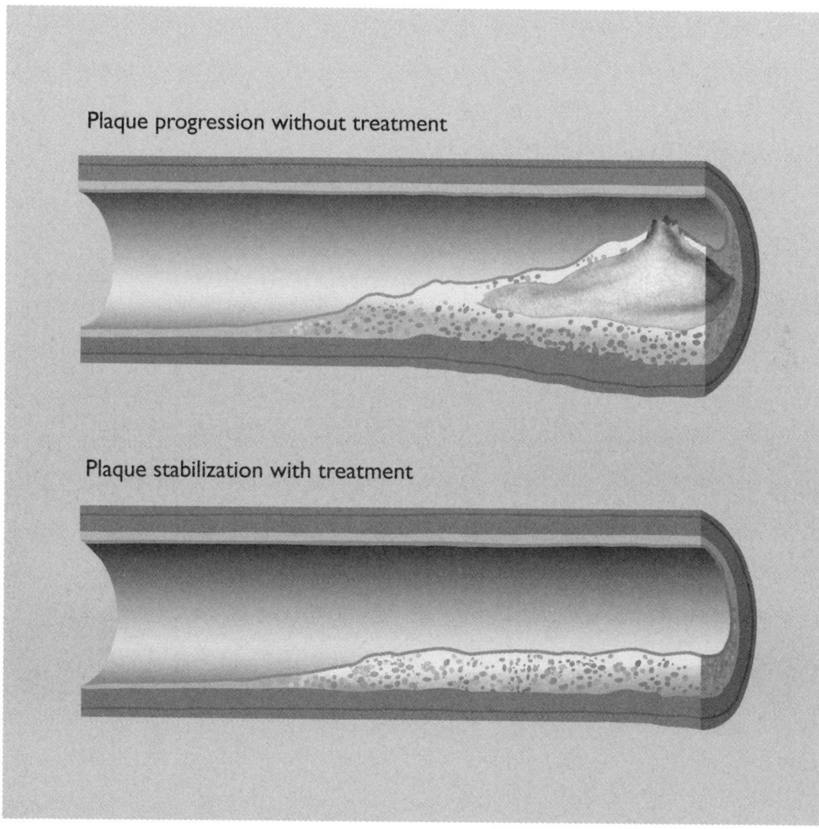

Chapter 4

MEASURING LIPIDS AND LIPOPROTEINS

LIKE MUCH OF MEDICINE, huge strides in understanding and treating lipid disorders have been made recently. Just 50 years ago, physicians discovered the importance of and focused their attention on the total cholesterol. We began to understand the significance of LDL-C in the '70s, HDL-C in the '80s, and inflammation, apoB, and lipoprotein particles in the '00s, and today non-HDL.

We routinely measure and treat the LDL-C. But evidence increasingly shows that cardiovascular risk is more directly proportional to the sum of all atherogenic cholesterol, which we know as non-HDL. Non-HDL is particularly important in the growing ranks of patients with the metabolic syndrome and type 2 diabetes.

Why Non-HDL-C is a better risk predictor and target of therapy than LDL-C

Non-HDL-C includes LDL-C (including IDL-C) plus cholesterol carried by TG-rich lipoprotein particles (VLDL-C and chylomicron cholesterol). VLDL-C is the largest component of triglyceride-rich lipoprotein cholesterol. The contribution from cholesterol carried in chylomicron particles and chylomicron remnants is minimal in the fasting state except in severe hypertriglyceridemia. Non-HDL-C may, for practical purposes, be considered to be the sum of cholesterol carried by LDL and VLDL particles.

Illustration 12 Non-HDL-C is the cholesterol carried by all apoB lipoproteins

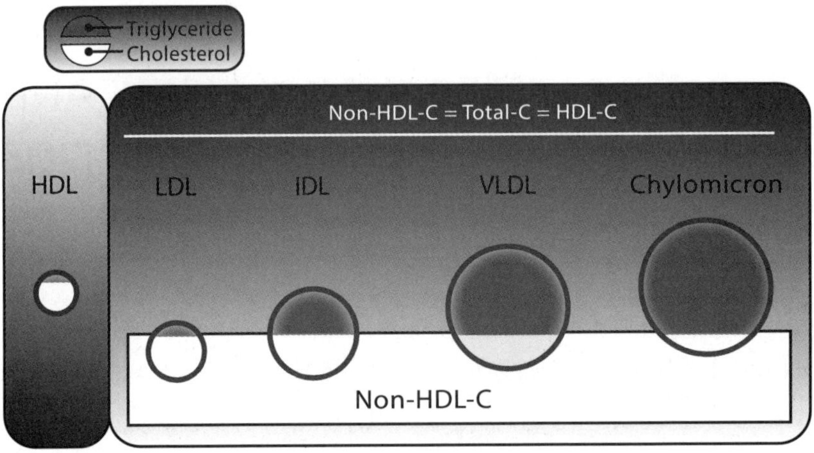

1. VLDL-C is at least as strongly associated with CVD event risk per mg/dL as is LDL-C, which explains the superiority of non-HDL-C over LDL-C as a predictor of cardiovascular event risk.
2. Elevated non-HDL-C due to increased VLDL-C is likely to be an important source of residual risk in a subgroup of statin-treated patients with well-controlled LDL-C.
3. Because VLDL-C is at least as atherogenic as LDL-C, non-HDL-C should be the preferred target of therapy.

Hitting target LDL-C and non-HDL-C—an improvement opportunity

Unfortunately, many people with lipid disorders have not yet been diagnosed and are not on treatment. In 2015, the CDC reported that between 1999 and 2012 the percentage of Americans with high cholesterol decreased from 18.3% to 12.9%. However, the same study notes that only 48% of adults with high cholesterol are on treatment to lower their LDL levels.

In 1993, NCEP ATP II further emphasized the importance of risk classification and the importance of both HDL-C and lifestyle. In 2001,

NCEP ATP III emphasized risk stratification with different risk categories, each with their own target goals for LDL-C and for non-HDL-C when the triglycerides exceed 200. These were updated in 2004 with the recognition of the optional benefit of even lower LDL-C targets in high- and very high-risk groups.

Unfortunately, recent studies show we still have substantial room for improvement. The 2005 NEPTUNE study (Davidson *Am J Card* 2005; 96: 556–563) shows that only 67% of 4,885 patients achieved their LDL cholesterol treatment goal and even fewer hit their non-HDL-C goal. The results were even worse for patients in the very high-risk categories.

Table 9 Percentage of patients meeting ATP III targets
(Davidson *Am J Card* 2005; 96: 556–563)

Risk Group	% reaching LDL-C goal	% reaching non-HDL-C goal
TG < 200		
0 – 1 risk factor	89	
≥ 2 risk factors	76	
CHD and CHD equivalents	57	
TG > 200		
0 – 1 risk factor		64
≥ 2 risk factors		52
CHD and CHD equivalents		27
Diabetes	40%	
CHD at very high risk	18%	

Dismal results were also found in a study of 41,000 high-risk patients with atherosclerosis all of whom were members of a quality managed care organization. "Among patients with an atherosclerosis diagnosis and CVD event, lipid-modifying therapy was received by [only] 50% before diagnosis and 57% after diagnosis, compared with 37% before and 48% after diagnosis for patients with an atherosclerosis diagnosis and no previous CVD event." (McKenny, J *Clin Lipid* 2009; 3: 385–392)

This data strongly suggests that even though we havestarted to lower the risk of CVD, we still have much work to do. Not every patient has been tested, not everyone with a lipid problem is treated to goal, and even people with atherosclerosis are not adequately treated. Patients need to know that preventive cardiology treatments do lower their risk of future events.

Everyone needs to have their lipids measured; EHRs should automatically calculate the patient's ten-year cardiovascular risk and print it on the discharge summary. Patients should know their ten-year risk and their LDL-C and non-HDLC goals just as they know they know that a blood pressure over 140/90 is too high. And every patient should be treated by guidelines to meet these goals. Then and only then will we continue to lower the appallingly high rate of CVD.

Fasting or non-fasting blood testing

A blood specimen is required to determine the difference between the patient's current LDL-C and non-HDL-C and their target goals according to the NCEP (see Chapter 9.)

Q: Must the patient be fasting?

A: The answer depends on what you are measuring. Eating raises plasma triglycerides but only has a minimal impact on total cholesterol or HDL-C or apo B. LDL-C is a calculated number that depends on the level of plasma triglycerides and therefore requires a fasting specimen. Non-HDL, however, does not require fasting.

Yes, the patient must be fasting if you want LDL-C. A fasting sample is required for the classic lipid profile (total cholesterol, triglycerides, HDL-C, and LDL-C) because the treatment goals and proven benefit of treatment are targeted at LDL-C.

But the patient need not fast if you want total cholesterol, HDL-C, non-HDL-C, direct LDL, or apo B. Total cholesterol and HDL are the only measurements you need to determine non-HDL-C.

Cholesterol

The total serum cholesterol, often abbreviated TC, is the sum of all of the cholesterol carried in all of the lipoproteins, including the cholesterol carried in both the atherogenic apo B lipoproteins (chylomicron remnants, VLDL + IDL + LDL + Lp(a)); and the usually anti-atherogenic apoA-1 lipoprotein (HDL).

TC = LDL-C + VLDL-C + IDL-C + Lp(a)-C + HDL-C

This chapter will look at clinically applicable measurements of total cholesterol, LDL-C, triglycerides, HDL-C, and at the measurements of lipoproteins.

Key points

- LDL-C becomes pathologic when it is somewhere above 50, the upper physiologic level required for biologic function.
- Under physiologic conditions, the LDL-C represents 90% of the atherogenic cholesterol in serum.
- Although all apo B-carrying lipoproteins can be atherogenic, in general, 90% of the pathologic cholesterol (the one that enters the vessel intima) is carried in the LDL-P. That explains why LDL-C is the primary NCEP target of treatment.
- Non-HDL cholesterol (non-HDL-C) is the cholesterol carried within all of the apo B-containing (potentially atherogenic) lipoproteins in a deciliter of plasma. Non-HDL-C equals TC – HDL-C.

Total cholesterol

Cholesterol has three main functions in the body: (1) cholesterol is essential to maintain cellular membranes and membrane enzyme activity; and, cholesterol is a precursor to both (2) steroid hormones and (3) bile salts.

With the notable exception of calculating the important non-HDL cholesterol, knowing a patient's total cholesterol does not provide much value.

LDL-C

Under normal metabolic conditions, LDL-C identifies the atherogenic cholesterol, because 90% of the atherogenic cholesterol is carried in LDL-P. This "normal metabolic condition" begins to fall apart as the triglyceride rises above a number somewhere between 100 and 150.

LDL-C is typically a calculated number. The Friedewald formula for calculating LDL-C is total cholesterol (TC) minus the sum of the cholesterol in HDL-P (HDL-C) and the cholesterol in VLDL-P (VLDL-C (or TG/5)). This calculation assumes that (1) all triglycerides are carried by the VLDL-P, and (2) that one-fifth of the VLDL-P is cholesterol and four-fifths of the VLDL-P is triglyceride. This formula works well when the triglycerides are under 150. See Chart 4 on page 115. However, as the triglycerides rise, the formula works less reliably until it is useless when the triglycerides exceed 400. And that happens because, as the triglycerides rise, the enzyme CETP exchanges triglycerides from the triglyceride-rich VLDL-P for cholesterol esters in both LDL-P and HDL-P.

Table 10 Friedewald equation when using mg/dL

LDL-C = TC – (HDL-C + VLDL-C)
or
LDL-C = TC – (HDL-C + TG/5)

Even though we now understand that it is the apo B lipoproteins that cause atherosclerosis, LDL-C remains the primary target of therapy because (1) the level of LDL-C is associated with the anatomic development of atherosclerosis, (2) multiple studies have shown that lowering LDL-C effectively produces a linear reduction in all coronary events, and (3) NCEP has spent 25 years promoting LDL-C as the primary target for therapy.

Triglycerides

The medical community has long relegated triglycerides to second-class citizenship, because the association of triglycerides with cardiovascular disease was difficult to prove. Many now see hypertriglyceridemia as a marker for other lipoprotein abnormalities that cause premature CVD. Increasingly, experts recognize that triglyceride levels between 150 and 500 increase the cardiovascular risk, particularly in patients with cardiometabolic disease, while triglycerides over 500 increase the risk of pancreatitis. Actually, the trigs of 500 themselves do not pose a risk of pancreatitis. Rather fasting trigs of 500 mean that the lipases are fully saturated, and any further increase in fatty acids as might occur after a fatty meal can easily send the trigs sky high—and that is when the pancreatitis appears.

Serum triglycerides are all of the triglycerides in plasma lipoproteins, which include any chylomicron remnants, VLDL, IDL, and even the triglyceride in LDL-P and HDL-P. Under optimal physiologic conditions, plasma triglycerides are in the 50 to 70 range, definitely < 100.

NCEP ATP III has the following criteria for triglycerides. Please note they define "high-risk" triglyceride levels as anything greater than 200.

Table 11 NCEP Classification of Triglyceride Levels from ATP III

Normal	< 100
Borderline	> 150
High risk	> 200
Very high risk	> 500

To help put the importance of triglycerides into perspective, we quote here from the 2002 NCEP ATP III:

> . . . elevations in serum triglycerides can be considered a marker for atherogenic remnant lipoproteins, for other lipid risk factors (small LDL particles and low HDL), for other non-lipid risk

> factors (elevated blood pressure), and for emerging risk factors (insulin resistance, glucose intolerance, prothrombotic state). Thus, the finding of elevated serum triglycerides helps to identify persons who are at risk and who need intervention for risk reduction. In addition, when triglyceride levels are ≥ 200 mg/dL, the presence of increased quantities of atherogenic remnant lipoproteins can heighten CHD risk substantially beyond that predicted by LDL cholesterol alone. For these reasons, ATP III modified the triglyceride classification to give more attention to moderate elevations. (*Circulation* 2002; p. 3168)

Triglycerides are at the center of the modern lipid disease: cardiometabolic disease with visceral obesity, insulin resistance, type 2 diabetes, hypertension, and the sedentary, high-carbohydrate lifestyle. The triglycerides themselves do not cause atherosclerosis, it is the company they keep (i.e., the cholesterol composition of the triglyceride-rich lipoproteins such as VLDL and VLDL remnants) that causes the trouble.

Non-HDL-C

Non-HDL-C includes all of the cholesterol in all of the potentially atherogenic lipoproteins containing apo B (any lingering chylomicron remnants, VLDL, IDL, LDL, and Lp(a)). Non-HDL does a better job of identifying atherosclerotic risk than does LDL.

It is calculated by subtracting the HDL-C from the TC. Non-HDL-C can—and should—be calculated on all standard lipid panels because it is superior to LDL for measuring the risk and is clinically useful in guiding more complete and accurate lipid management. Non-HDL does not require fasting.

The calculated non-HDL can be thought of as a cheap and often adequate surrogate for direct measurements of LDL-P and apo B.

Non-HDL-C is useful when the triglycerides are in the 200 to 499 range, because this level increases the activity of CETP, which moves the cholesterol ester from LDL-P and HDL-P to VLDL-P. This increases the cholesterol concentration in the now more atherogenic VLDL-P and IDL-P and decreases the amount of cholesterol carried by each LDL-P. But, as noted previously, non-HDL-C cannot be calculated when the triglycerides exceed 500.

Apo B

It is possible, and often desirable, to measure serum levels of apo B, because apo B particles attach to and carry cholesterol into the intima, starting the process of cardiovascular disease. Apo B has four major advantages over LDL-C: (1) serum apo B measurements are superior to LDL-C for the identification of cardiovascular risk, (2) serum apo B includes all of the potentially atherogenic lipoproteins, (3) each atherogenic lipoprotein carries only one apo B, and (4) a serum apo B does not require fasting. The apo B particles are those that directly deliver cholesterol ester into the arterial intima. The risk of cardiovascular disease is more clearly related to the levels of apo B or LDL-P than the LDL-C. See Chart 5 on page 130.

Testing levels of apo B is more common in Canada than in the US, but is gaining ground here with improvements in testing protocols and availability of the testing laboratories.

Data from the JUPITER trial shows the discordance between LDL-C, non-HDL-C, and apo B.

Table 12 Baseline lipids in the JUPITER trial compared to the population percentiles from the Framingham Offspring Study (Sniderman at the Second Annual Preventive Cardiology Summit of the University of Chicago, April 18, 2009)

		Population percentiles from FOS	
	Baseline JUPITER data In mg/dL	Males	Females
LDL-C	108	23	30
Non-HDL-C	137	25	40
Apo B	109	60	70

Lipoprotein testing

Knowing the plasma level of the various lipoproteins is sometimes more important than knowing the plasma level of LDL-C or non-HDL-C when trying to prevent cardiovascular disease. Clinical labs now offer testing for lipoprotein particle number. Recent studies show that understanding lipoprotein particle number is important for optimizing lipid management. Lipoprotein abnormalities and discordance between the LDL-C and the LDL-P are most marked in patients with cardiometabolic disease—and sometimes those with even a whiff of cardiometabolic disease. This is explored further in Chapter 8.

Intuitively, it would seem that we could optimize treatment of lipid disorders by treating LDL-C, non-HDL-C, LDL-P, and apo B to the same target percentile. These are shown in the table below. However, treating the apo B to less than the 20th percentile and the non-HDL-C to less than the 10th percentile often requires three medications. At this point, the scientific evidence does not justify the risks involved with such an aggressive treatment.

Table 13 Distribution of lipids in Framingham Offspring Study
adapted from Contois JH *Clin Chem* 2009;407-419

Percentile	LDL-C	Non-HDL-C	LDL-P	Apo B
2	70	83	720	54
10	88	104	940	69
20	100	119	1100	78
50	130	153	1440	97
80	160	187	1820	118
90	176	205	2020	130
95	191	224	2210	140

Risk assessment and treatment targets

So the question remains, what is the best target for therapy? Is it LDL-C or LDL-P or apo B or non-HDL or triglycerides? Every clinical outcome studies has confirmed that lowering LDL-C reduces the risk of coronary vascular disease.

The LDL-C is a standard finding on all lipid reports and is the primary treatment target of all guidelines. A large number of randomized, controlled trials have shown that lowering LDL-C will lower coronary events. The 2004 Update of the NCEP ATP III (*Circ* 2004; 110: 227–239) states that "for every 30-mg/dL change in LDL-C, the relative risk for CHD is changed in proportion by about 30%." The Heart Protection Study showed that this one-to-one relationship held even for people with a starting LDL-C below 100. This is reinforced by the Clinical Cholesterol Trialists who showed that for every mmol (40 mg/dl) reduction in LDL, the risk of a major cardiovascular event fell by 25%, and there is no lower limit to this ratio.

Increasingly non-HDL is recognized as the primary target of therapy, because it is more strongly related to the risk of ASCVD in patients with both normal and elevated triglycerides.

Steps to optimal lipid management

When treating a patient with lipid or cardiovascular disorders, the following steps can guide you to maximal clinical benefit. We will go over these in much more detail in Chapter 8.

1. Treat triglycerides over 500.
2. Identify high-risk patients, and for the remainder, calculate their ten-year cardiovascular risk.
3. Treat with the correct intensity statin as written in the 2013 ACC/AHA guidelines.
4. Know the corresponding patient's LDL and non-HDL-C goals as per the guidelines of the NLA or 2004 NCEP update.
5. Treat the patient to their LDL-C and non-HDL-C goals.

Ensuring that the non-HDL and lipoproteins also at goal is doubly important in patients with cardiometabolic risk (obesity, insulin resistance, pre-diabetes, impaired fasting glucose, diabetes, or hypertriglyceridemia), because LDL-C, apo B, non-HDL, and LDL-P are likely to be discordant in these patients. This is the area where residual risk (the risk remaining after the patient is treated to LDL-C goal) is likely to be greatest. Think of it this way: our most common statin treatments lower the risk of CVD by 30%, which means that our patients are still exposed to 70% of their pre-treatment risk.

Section II

The Genetics and Medical Conditions That Cause Lipid Disorders

Chapter 5

Inherited Lipid Disease

Lipidology lacks a single, clear, unifying classification of the many lipid disorders. In 2015, we continue to use a 65-year-old classification as the starting place to define inherited lipid diseases, one that does not include recently recognized genetic diseases. Some experts classify lipid disorders as disorders of either catabolism or metabolism. Most practitioners use the "see-it, treat-it" method of addressing lipid problems.

This chapter will identify the major inherited lipid disorders. Correct identification of the disorder or disease is the all-important first step to an organized treatment approach.

Key Points

- Familial lipid diseases require early identification of both the patient and the family members.
- Lipid disorders are either entirely inherited (e.g., familial hypercholesterolemia is an inherited disorder of the LDL-Receptor) or an inherited condition exacerbated by environmental factors (e.g., familial combined hypercholesterolemia is an over-production of apo B lipoproteins exacerbated by the development of insulin resistance).

Fredrickson classification system

In 1965, Fredrickson proposed a classification of lipid disorders. We still refer to and use this classification method. Understanding this chart will help you understand what and why you are choosing one medication over another or whether you need to test family members.

Unfortunately, the Fredrickson system has at least two deficiencies. First, it is incomplete because it does not include the more recently discovered genetic disorders (e.g., genetically low HDL). And confusingly, many patients with hypertriglyceridemia can be either type IIb, IV, or sometimes even V.

In a given patient, this Fredrickson classification holds most true for type I or hyperchylomicronemia and type IIa familial hypercholesterolemia. For all other classifications, the serum of a single patient can move from one category to another depending on environmental factors or treatment, because the level of enzyme activity can be increased or decreased depending on the clinical milieu.

Table 14 Fredrickson Classification Types

I	Common name	Hyperchylomicronemia
	TC:TG	TG usually > 1000 TC = 1/10 of TG
	Metabolic problem	Deficiency of LPL or apo C-II
	Clinical presentation	Often seen in children with TG > 1000 Chylomicrons in overnight serum Eruptive xanthomas and recurrent pancreatitis Low atherogenicity
	Frequency	1 in 1,000,000
IIa	**Common name**	**Familial hypercholesterolemia FH**
	TC:TG	LDL 180 to 350 in HeFH LDL 350 to 600 in HoFH TG normal
	Inheritance	Autosomal dominant
	Metabolic problem	Defective LDL-R or defective apo B or gain of function of PCSK9

	Clinical presentation	Severe hypercholesterolemia Early CAD Autosomal dominant Tendon xanthomas, xanthelasmas, corneal arcus
	Frequency in gen pop	Homozygous 1/1,000,000 Heterozygous 1/500 with worldwide distribution
	Frequency in lipid clinic	10%
	Note	FH is under-diagnosed. Making the correct diagnosis and aggressive family testing is the only proven way to identify and treat this potentially fatal disease.
IIb	**Common name**	**Familial combined hypercholesterolemia FCH**
	TC:TG	TC 200 to 400 TG 150 to 500 HDL usually low
	Inheritance	Autosomal dominant Also induced or promoted by the metabolic syndrome
	Metabolic problem	Hepatic over-production of apo B leading to increased plasma VLDL
	Clinical presentation	Premature CAD out of proportion to modest degree of hyperlipidemia Lots of small, dense LDL-P Apo B > LDL-C Commonly seen with insulin resistance and metabolic syndrome Does not have xanthomas
	Frequency in gen pop	1/200
	Frequency in lipid clinic	> 40%
III	**Common name**	**Dysbetalipoproteinemia**
	TC:TG	TC 300 TG 300
	Metabolic problem	Apo E2/E2 because E2/E2 does not bind with LDL-R (aka LDL-R = B/E receptor)

	Clinical presentation	IDL (VLDL remnants) are increased Tubero-eruptive xanthomas on elbows and knees Orange palmar xanthomas
	Frequency	Rare
IV	**Common name**	**Familial hypertriglyceridemia**
	TC:TG	TC 250 TG 400 to 1000
	Inheritance	Autosomal dominant
	Metabolic problem	Impaired lipolysis of TG (impaired LPL, or inherited decrease of apoC II or increase of apoC III) or increased production of VLDL
	Clinical presentation	Family history of hypertriglyceridemia Exacerbated by high carbohydrate diets and/or alcohol Low atherogenicity
	Frequency in gen pop	Common
	Frequency in lipid clinic	> 40%
V	**Common name**	**Familial lipoprotein lipase deficiency**
	TC:TG	TC 250 TG 1000 and up
	Metabolic problem	Lipoprotein Lipase Deficiency Both chylomicrons and triglycerides present
	Clinical presentation	Presents in adulthood, often with obesity, diabetes, and metabolic syndrome
	Frequency in gen pop	Uncommon

Other non-Fredrickson inherited lipid diseases and conditions

Several inherited lipid diseases have been identified since the Fredrickson classification table was written. These include Lp(a), inherited low HDL levels, high remnant levels, and siterosterolemia—and the fortuitously inherited low LDL levels. Undoubtedly, more research will lead to more lipid disorders ascribed to inherited or genetic enzyme deficiencies.

Lp(a)

Lp(a) is an apoB lipoprotein with an apoA attached. Inherited in an autosomal dominant fashion, Lp(a) is an independent risk factor for CVD. An elevated level of Lp(a) is doubly bad because: (1) it is atherogenic like LDL and (2) it is pro-thrombotic because of its similarity to plasminogen. Elevated levels of Lp(a) are particularly common in South Asians and may account for their early and aggressive CAD.

Inherited low HDL

Inherited low HDL has four causes, three that may be or are associated with premature CVD: (1) familial hypo-alpha-lipoproteinemia; (2) inherited deficiency of ABCA-1; (3) a deficiency of LCAT; and one that is cardioprotective: (4) HDL-Milano.

Autosomal dominant familial hypo-alpha-lipoproteinemia is a common inherited cause of a low HDL. You should suspect the diagnosis if the HDL-C is low and the apo B or LDL-P numbers are normal (which is to say that insulin resistance is not the cause of the low HDL-C). Familial hypo-alpha lipoproteinemia is associated with increased CVD risk.

The next two causes of low HDL are distinctly rare. Both are disorders of enzymes that move cholesterol from macrophages to apo A-1, the start of the important reverse cholesterol transport process. One is Tangier Disease, an inherited absence of ABCA-1. This absence limits the body's ability to transfer cholesterol from a macrophage to nascent apo A-1 (the first step of turning apo A-1 into an HDL lipoprotein). The patient's tissues fill with cholesterol because it cannot be moved back into circulation. The patients have hepatosplenomegaly and premature CAD. The second rare cause of low HDL is heterozygote LCAT deficiency, where the missing enzyme is responsible for esterifying cholesterol of the apo A-1, leaving the HDL incompletely developed. Heterozygotes have corneal opacities and early CAD.

And, the very interesting HDL-Milano: an HDL-P that is highly protective even at very low plasma levels—but tragically rare. This highly unusual HDL-P originated from a single couple in eighteenth-century Limone sul Garda, Italy. It is an inherited low HDL that is associated with a very low risk of coronary artery disease, because HDL-Milano is a highly efficient reverse cholesterol transporter.

- Be aware: Most low HDL-C is not inherited. Far and away the most common cause of low HDL-C is the pandemic of obesity, inactivity, and a standard American diet. Other causes include a very low-fat diet and the use of anabolic steroids.

Inherited elevated HDL

There are several inherited causes of elevated HDL. The first, seen almost exclusively in people of Japanese ancestry, is an inherited loss-of-function mutation in the alleles for the gene that encodes CETP. This mutation increases the concentration of cholesterol-rich HDL-P, which are too large to be efficiently catabolized. Other enzyme deficiencies that increase HDL include hepatic lipase deficiency and defective SRB1. And lastly is primary hyperalphalipoproteinemia, the basket into which we put everything else.

Inherited low LDL-C

Some patients have inherited low levels of LDL-C. These patients may be heterozygotes for hypo-beta-lipoproteinemia. Homozygotes cannot carry cholesterol to cells for membrane formation and do not survive. Heterozygotes were discussed in Chapter 1 as part of the discussion of how low can LDL-C safely go. Other causes of low LDL include inherited mutations in PCSK9 and NPC1L1.

Inherited increased absorption of phytosterols

The other inherited disorder that causes premature CAD is sitosterolemia or phytosterolemia. It is a very rare (< 100 diagnosed cases, although probably under-diagnosed) autosomal-recessive lipid disorder characterized by increased absorption of the plant sterols campesterol and sitosterol and various plant stanols. Or, to be more precise, the disease is the inherited loss of the ability to excrete plant sterols and stanols from the intestinal enterocyte directly back into the intestine. This mutation lies in the ABCG-5 and

ABCG-8 transporter enzymes, which pump the sterols and stanols from the enterocyte back into the intestine.

The CVD in these patients is actually caused by the increased systemic levels of phytosterols, which are highly toxic to cells. Patients with siterosterolemia also have elevated LDL-C because the LDL-Rs are down-regulated. These patients present looking like classic familial hypercholesterolemia with tendon xanthomas, arcus senilis, and premature coronary vascular disease.

Chapter 6

FAMILIAL HYPERCHOLESTEROLEMIA

We are devoting an entire chapter to the inherited disease Familial Hypercholesterolemia (FH) because 1) it is the leading cause of inherited premature death worldwide; 2) preventive treatment is available, inexpensive and effective; but 3) sadly the diagnosis is made and effective treatment given less than 20% of the time.

This disease is low-hanging fruit. We can and must do better. We need to diagnosis and treat this disease at young ages to prevent atherosclerosis. So let's start to better understand this very real disease.

FH is an inherited autosomal dominant disease with complete penetrance. It is characterized by an LDL that is twice normal from birth and early onset of atherosclerosis. Untreated, clinically apparent atherosclerosis develops by age 55 in males and age 65 in females. The WHO estimates that only 20% of people with FH reach the age of 70. You can't say it much clearer than the University of Utah FH Program, which entitles their FH program MEDPED–Make Early Diagnosis to Prevent Early Deaths.

In FH, the predominate defect is in the LDL-Receptor with the result that LDL-P are inefficiently removed from circulation. Ninety-five percent of the 1,600 known mutations are in the LDL-R, with the remainder being a gain of function mutation of PCSK9 or mutations in apoB. In all genetic mutations, the result is that LDL-P are not removed efficiently from the circulation and circulate for three to five days, in contrast to the more normal day and a half. The result is a phenotype where the LDL-C is twice normal—from birth onward.

This disease is incredibly common. Worldwide one in 250 to one in 500 people carry one mutation (heterozygotes) and one in a 500,000 are homozygous. Every practice in the world has at least a couple of these heterozygous patients. And half of all of their first-degree relatives will also carry the gene and need to be identified and treated.

Patients with FH must be identified and treated based on their LDL-C elevations because they have a lifetime elevation of LDL that markedly increases their risk of a premature heart attack. The problem is the long, silent latency period, or by the time, we make the diagnosis in adulthood, the patient often has advanced atherosclerosis.

Here is the all-too-common way these patients present to the lipidologist: A 52-year-old presents with a STEMI and the cardiac cath shows advanced atherosclerosis. His LDL is 225, and he tells you it has been "way over 200" his entire life. He tried statins once or twice, but his physician never made a diagnosis or emphasized the severity of his disease or the importance of statins. The patient felt well so he did not renew the prescriptions. We have both seen patients who have routine physicals with lipid panels showing an LDL of 225 who were not even offered treatment.

Untreated FH causes a huge amount of premature disease. If we do not identify these patients and treat them, half of these male patients will have a heart attack before the age of 55 and half of females will have a heart attack before age 65. Those are awful numbers.

People with FH just have different LDL-C than normal patients. Their LDL-C ranges from 180 to 350. The triglycerides are usually normal. Remember they basically have half of the LDL-R, which gives them twice the circulating LDL-C. The illustration 13 below shows this clearly. The cutpoint of LDL-C between the normal and FH is 190 (5 mmol). Certainly not everyone with an LDL of 190 will have FH, but that is the cutpoint at which you seriously have to ask the question.

Illustration 13 Distribution of LDL in normal and FH patients

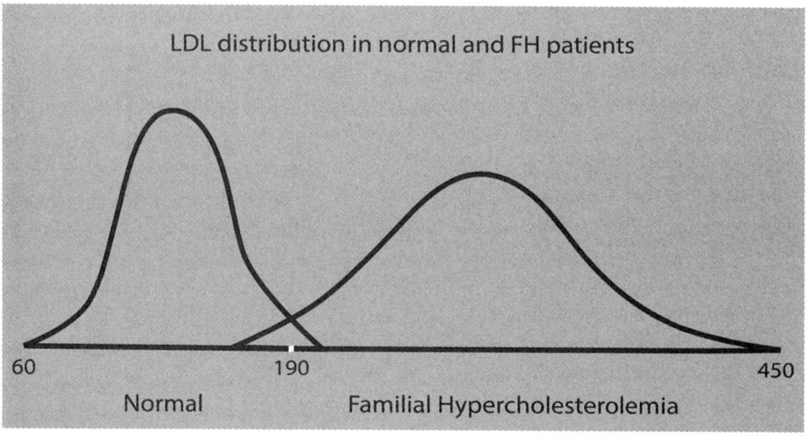

So who are these people? How do we identify them? Unfortunately, there are a couple of answers, but no one single diagnostic criteria that works best in clinic. The criteria for research have poor sensitivity and specificity in the clinic. Fewer than half of the patients with FH will have the clinical xanthomas which are so diagnostic of the disease (see photos below). Genetic testing has a large percentage of false negatives, and some with positive tests have lipid levels that are elevated but below classic cutpoints of 190.

Illustration 14 Photos of Achilles tendon xanthomas. Xanthelasmas of the eyelid, and extensor tendon xanthomas

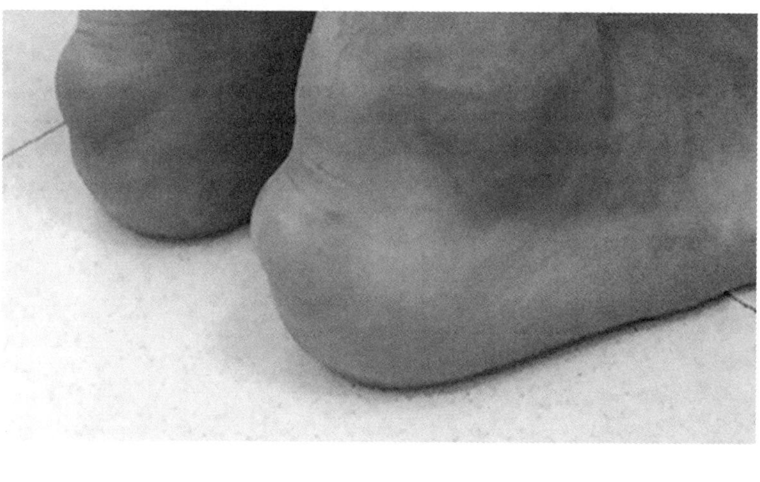

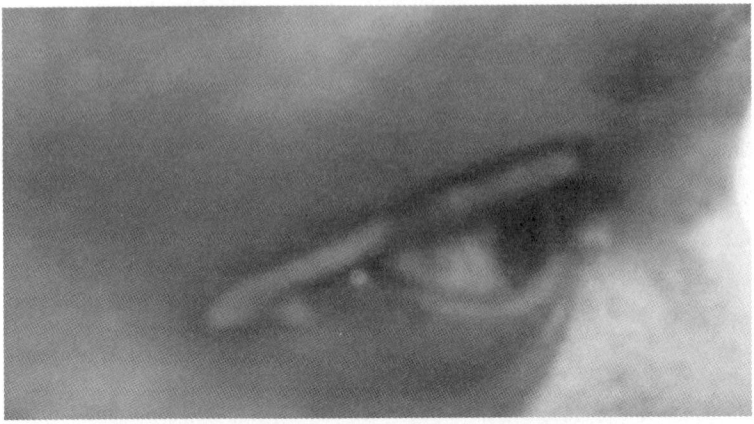

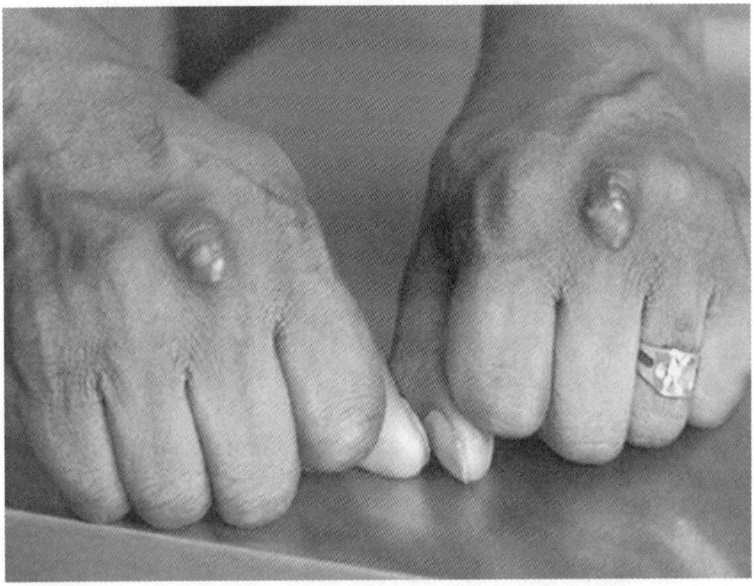

The Dutch Lipid Criteria (shown in Table 15 below) nicely includes and highlights the important diagnostic features of familial hypercholesterolemia. And it is easy to follow. The authors highly recommend its use.

Table 15 Dutch Lipid Clinic Criteria for Familial Hypercholesterolemia

Definite	> 8
Probable	6 to 8
Possible	3 to 5
Unlikely	1 or 2

Family history	Points
▸ Coronary or vascular disease in a first-degree relative (M < 55, F < 60) or ▸ First-degree relative with LDL > 190	1
▸ First-degree relative with tendinous xanthoma or arcus cornealis or ▸ Children < 18 with LDL > 95th percentile	2
Clinical history	
▸ Patient with premature CAD	2
▸ Patient with premature cerebral or peripheral vascular disease	1
Physical exam	
▸ Tendinous xanthoma	6
▸ Arcus cornealis < age 45	4
LDL level	
▸ > 330 (8.5 mmol)	8
▸ 250 to 329 (6.25 to 8.5)	5
▸ 190 to 249 (4.75 to 6.26)	3
▸ 160 to 189 (4 to 4.75)	1
DNA analysis	
▸ Functional mutation in LDL-R, apoB, or PCSK9	8

Alternatively, the Simon Broome Criteria can be used to diagnose both definite and probable FH.

Table 16 Simon Broome Criteria for Diagnosing FH

Definite FH	Adult TC > 300 or LDL > 190 Child TC > 260 or LDL > 160	Plus tendon xanthomas in the patient or a first-degree relative
	Genetic test for LDL-R, PCSK9, or apoB mutation	
Probable FH	Adult TC > 300 or LDL > 190 Child TC > 260 or LDL > 160	Plus family history of MI < age 60 in first-degree or < age 50 in second-degree relative

Although genetic testing is commonly done in the EU, it is uncommon in America because of false positives and false negatives. The authors rarely use genetic testing in their preventive cardiology clinics.

In an effort to promote earlier diagnosis, the authors would like to promote the simple definition:

> Diagnose FH when the LDL > 190 plus either xanthomas or a first-degree relative with premature heart disease, with elevated LDL-C (may be on treatment), or xanthomas.

We need remember that an LDL of 160 to 190 is elevated but does not mean that we must jump to the diagnosis of FH. This range is the top quintile of the normal LDL distribution. Also included in this group are the many people with hypothyroidism, renal or hepatic disease, or the any of the multitude of reasons that an LDL can rise (see page 72).

Once you make the diagnosis of FH, you are obligated to tell the patient four things: 1) he or she has a serious, life-threatening disease, 2) effective treatment is available that can lower their risk to normal 3) only if he takes the medication and follows a heart-healthful lifestyle forever, and 4) that all first-degree relatives must be tested (including children) and treated if they also carry the mutation.

The diagnosis of FH in children varies by their age and expected 95th percentile of the LDL level. In general, if the parent has the disease and a child has an LDL > 140, they have a > 95% chance of also having FH—and potentially needing statin treatment starting in early adolescence and definitely by age 20.

There is some disagreement about when or whether to treat children and adolescents with heterozygous FH. In general, children under age 12 are treated with aggressive lifestyle modification. Some experts begin using statins at age 12 with a target LDL of 130 (3.5 mmol). The CHARON study with 196 children showed statins were well tolerated with no change in growth and sexual maturation. But all specialists agree that all patients with FH should be started on treatment by the age of 20.

Having identified these patients with FH, when and how do we treat them?

Obviously, the first step is a heart-healthful lifestyle: Once again follow the AHA Simple Seven. Avoid tobacco smoke in all its forms (first- and second-hand and e-cigarettes), get daily activity or exercise, do not be obese, and eat a heart-healthful diet that avoids junk and processed foods and emphasizes heart-healthy foods like olive oil, nuts, red berries, steel cut oatmeal, fish, and lots of fruits and veggies. Then closely monitor and treat blood pressure, blood sugar, and all diseases that increase inflammation.

However, even the most aggressive diet restrictions will not normalize LDL in patients with FH, not even close.

All heterozygous adult FH patients over the age 18 will need medication to lower their LDL enough to prevent premature CAD. Guidelines for primary prevention call for a > 50% reduction with an LDL target of < 100 (2.5 mmol). If secondary prevention, then the target is < 70 (1.8 mmol).

The only statins that have the power to lower LDL by > 50% are atorva 40 or 80 mg and rosuva 20 or 40 mg. Often additional medications are required. The authors often add ezetimibe, because it is well tolerated and lowers LDL by an additional 20%. Alternatively bile acid sequestrants may also be used, some of which are helpful in FH patients who also have type 2 diabetes.

Early and aggressive treatment is necessary to reduce the lifetime burden of atherogenic LDL in these patients. But, if treated early and aggressively enough, FH patients have a normal life expectancy as shown on the table below.

Chart 2 Statins signicantly improve CHD-free survival in FH

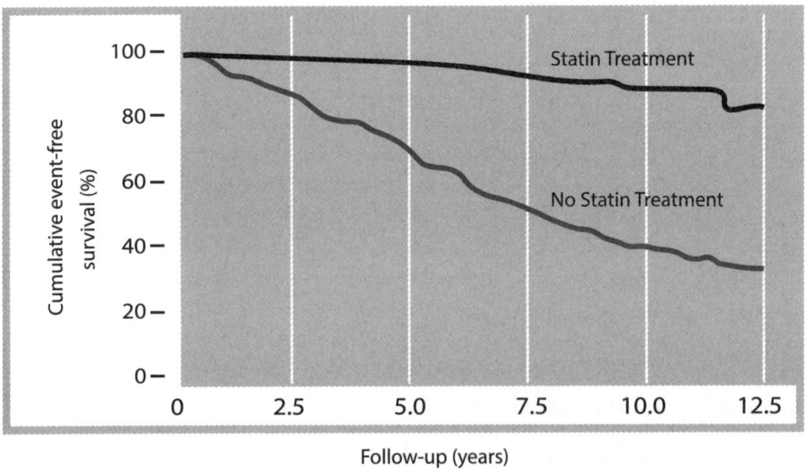

Versmissen, JBMJ 2008;337 :a2423

Many FH patients may not reach goal even with maximal therapy and a heart-healthful diet. These patients are candidates for the addition of the new PCSK9 inhibitors. As of this writing, two PCSK9 inhibitors have been approved: alirocumab (Praluent) and evolocumab (Repatha). They were FDA approved based on consistent positive results from Phase 3 trials: ODYSSEY for alirocumab and OSLER for evolocumab. The outcome data from these trials will be published in 2017. More on these medications in the chapter on medications.

Some FH patients will need be referred to a tertiary medical center. These include heterozygous FH patients who are intolerant of statins, FH patients who have had an event or have multiple risk factors, or cannot otherwise reach goal, and all patients with homozygous FH. These patients may be candidates for the PCSK9 inhibitors or rarely advanced therapies like apheresis or the orphan medications lomitapide and mipomersen.

In summary, when you see a patient with an LDL-C > 190 (4.5 mmol) in an adult or > 160 in an adolescent, use this checklist:

- ☐ Think FH until proven otherwise.
- ☐ Exclude other causes of elevated LDL-C (especially hypothyroidism).
- ☐ Ask about family history of premature CAD including events, stents, and cholesterol lowering medications.
- ☐ Look for xanthomas in the patient and ask about family members who might have same.
- ☐ Use the diagnosis of LDL > 190 + FH of early disease or xanthomas to make diagnosis.
- ☐ If you make the diagnosis of FH, immediately start with both lifestyle and treat (unless pregnant) with atorva 40 or 80 or rosuva 20 or 40. Do not delay, even the most rigorous diets simply won't work.
- ☐ Tell patient that all first-degree relatives are at risk of having the same mutation. They all need a lipid test. In our clinics, we require that the patients bring us copies of the family's labs to be certain they were tested.
- ☐ Emphasize to the patient this treatment is for lifetime, because it is the only way to ensure a long life.

Chapter 7

Diseases and Drugs that Cause Lipid Abnormalities

In clinical practice, most lipid disorders are a combination of an underlying lipid disorder exacerbated by a medical condition or lifestyle choices, e.g., excess dietary carbohydrates, fats, or alcohol. The following lists identify medical conditions, diseases, or medications that you should consider when seeing a patient with lipid abnormalities. You should address these medical conditions and medications before you treat the lipid abnormality.

Key points

- Many common diseases, medical conditions, and medications exacerbate underlying lipid abnormalities, sometimes to an astonishing degree.
- The underlying medical disease or condition should be addressed before the lipid disorder is treated.
- Medication and supplement or herb lists should be reviewed and, if necessary, adjusted before lipid treatment is implemented.

Increased LDL-C

Seven diseases and one common condition raise LDL-C

There are seven medical conditions that raise LDL-C. You should always think about these in a patient with elevated LDL-C, particularly if the patient presents with a sudden increase in his or her LDL-C.

1. Hypothyroidism

   This is the most common medical condition that raises the LDL. Every patient with an LDL over 160 should have a TSH to look for hypothyroidism. If hypothyroid, correct the thyroid before treating the LDL.

2. Renal disease

   Do not get fooled here—check the urine for blood or protein. You are looking for new onset renal disease like nephrotic syndrome.

3. Obstructive liver disease

   See renal disease above, only think liver.

4. Anorexia nervosa

5. HIV both by itself and exacerbated by HAART

   It won't be the first time that someone suspected HIV because of a new increase in LDL-C.

6. Cushing syndrome

   Self evident if you consider the possibility.

7. Polycystic ovarian syndrome

   Be a hero: be the first to make the diagnosis and get the young lady the treatment she needs.

8. And the very normal condition: pregnancy

   If you, as a lipid doc, are the first to suspect pregnancy, then she and her other physicians have other issues to deal with.

9. Menopause

   Menopause will increase the LDL an average of 10%. Sometimes more.

Medications that raise LDL-C

Six common medications that raise LDL.

1. Anabolic steroids

   Anabolic steroids used for body building raise LDL and lower HDL. Steroids used therapeutically do not increase LDL.

2. Cyclosporines

   Many transplant patients are now moving back to the primary care offices for long-term care, but they still have the problems associated with transplant medications including elevated LDL.

3. Progestins (some, not all)

4. Thiazides

5. Fibrates if the initial triglyceride is significantly elevated

6. Prescription omega-3 if triglyceride is elevated

   Remember these last two every time you start a fibrate or omega-3 to lower significantly elevated triglycerides. You'll look like a wise clinician if you predict the rise in LDL-C, but you'll look even wiser if also predict that the Apo B will go down.

One medical condition that lowers LDL-C

1. An acute coronary syndrome

   The LDL-C falls within 24 hours of an acute coronary syndrome and does not return to baseline for 4 to 6 weeks. This is important to remember when you are called to treat lipid abnormalities in a patient with a recent coronary syndrome. Always use lipid values drawn within 24 hours of the MI to establish the baseline.

Increased triglycerides

Medical conditions that raise triglycerides

Two common medical conditions cause hypertriglyceridemia.

1. Far and away, the most common cause of elevated triglycerides is the current pandemic of insulin resistance, obesity, inactivity, and either a low-fat or a high-carbohydrate diet. Sometimes just a high-carbohydrate diet is enough to raise the trigs.
2. Alcohol excess

Eight diseases and one condition that cause a high triglyceride

There are eight primary diseases and one common condition that raise triglycerides.

1. Hypothyroidism

   Hypothyroidism impairs the functioning of lipoprotein lipase, which is important for the hydrolysis of chylomicrons and VLDL.

2. Poorly controlled diabetes mellitus

   An elevated A1C is associated with defects of lipoprotein lipase, which is important for the hydrolysis of chylomicrons and VLDL.

3. Type 1 Diabetes

   Triglycerides rise because insulin is not available to inhibit the adipose tissue hormone-sensitive lipase. This means that the insulin-sensitive lipase in adipose tissue is not turned off, and the adipocytes continue to pump out free fatty acids which are packaged with apo B in the liver and secreted as VLDL.

4. Type 2 Diabetes

   The cause of the hypertriglyceridemia in type 2 diabetics is a bit more complicated. The insulin resistance means that insulin is not available to shut off the hormone sensitive lipase, so the adipocytes increase their output of free fatty acids, which flood the liver, which in turn packages them with Apo B to make VLDL. Type 2 diabetes then has two major problems that both increase triglycerides: first is a hepatic over-production of VLDL in response to the increased FFA output from adipocytes, and second is a decreased function of LPL (lipoprotein lipase whose duty is to hydrolyze the triglycerides in VLDL) and an increase of apo C-III (whose function is to stop LPL).

5. Anorexia nervosa

   Lipodystrophy can be seen in this condition

6. HIV

   Lipodystrophy can also be seen in this condition.

7. Gaucher's

8. Hepatitis

9. Chronic renal disease

10. Pregnancy

Twelve medications that raise triglycerides

1. Bile acid sequestrants

   All bile acid sequestrants (used to lower LDL-C) can increase the triglyceride level when the starting triglycerides are elevated. They should all be used cautiously when the starting triglycerides exceed 300 and avoided when the trigs exceed 500.

2. Estrogens

   Estrogens have a complex effect on lipids. On the good side, they lower LDL, lower Lp(a), and increase HDL by 20%; but on the bad side, they raise TG, increase clotting mechanisms and activate metalloproteinases (which weaken atherosclerotic plaques making a plaque rupture more likely). Estrogens increase triglycerides by both stimulating hepatic production of VLDL and inhibiting hepatic lipase.

   Interestingly, estrogen patches do not raise triglycerides because they have a hepatic second pass through.

3. Oral contraceptives containing second-generation progestins

4. The SERMs (selective estrogen receptor modulators) tamoxifen, raloxifene, and clomiphene

   The SERMs may cause hypertriglyceridemia. Interestingly, they may also reduce LDL-C and Lp(a).

5. β-blockers

   β-blockers raise TG to a minor degree. In the Helsinki Heart Study, patients treated with beta blockers had a lower incidence of CHD despite slightly worse triglycerides.

6. Thiazide diuretics in high doses

7. Cyclosporine

   Cyclosporine increases triglycerides, LDL, and the serum concentration of all statins, although cyclosporine impacts fluvastatin the least.

8. Retinoids

9. Atypical anti-psychotics, particularly clozapine and olanzapine

10. Steroids

11. Protease inhibitors

12. Long-term interferon treatment

HDL-C

Five medications and two substances that lower HDL

1. Beta blockers, although not enough to increase mortality

2. Isoretinoids

3. Adding a glitazone to a fibrate

   Adding a glitazone to a fibrate may lower HDL significantly, although this is reported to happen only rarely.

4. Progestins

5. Anabolic steroids

   Anabolic steroids if used for weight training. The HDL-lowering effect of steroids is not seen with transdermal androgens or if the testosterone is used to treat hypogonadism.

6. Trans-fats

7. Smoking

Four medical conditions that cause a low HDL-C

1. Insulin resistance

   Far and away, the most common cause of a low HDL-C is the insulin resistance associated with our current pandemic of inactivity, obesity, and a high-carbohydrate diet.

2. Smoking

   The most common habit associated with a low HDL is tobacco. Quitting cigarettes can raise HDL by 20% within 8 weeks.

3. A high-carbohydrate diet
4. A very low-fat diet

A medical condition that raises HDL-C

1. Aerobic exercise

A medication and a chemical that raise HDL-C

1. Alcohol
2. Estrogens

SECTION III

Treatment Guidelines and Lipid Medications

Chapter 8
GUIDELINES

Lipid-treatment guidelines to lower the risk of heart disease have been in place for 30 years. For many years and in most countries, the lipid guidelines focused on lowering the LDL-C with treatment targets proportional to the patient's risk of CAD. Currently these include the guidelines of the National Lipid Association and most international guidelines (Canadian, European Society of Cardiology, the International Atherosclerosis Society, and the NICE guidelines of the UK). The current exception is that of the 2013 American Heart Association American College of Cardiology, which focuses primarily on matching the intensity of the statin treatment with the patient's risk and does not set specific LDL goals. Take your pick, in the main they will get to about the same place for those patients who need treatment—the important point is to start treatment for those patients with an increased ten-year risk of CAD.

Guidelines for the identification and treatment of lipid abnormalities have been in place since November 1985, when the National Heart, Lung, and Blood Institute (NHLBI) launched the National Cholesterol Education Program (NCEP). The goal of the program was to reduce atherosclerotic disease and death by reducing the number of Americans with high blood cholesterol. NCEP was based largely on the 1984 Lipid Research Clinics

Coronary Primary Prevention Trial, which showed that lowering serum cholesterol levels (even with a bile acid sequestrant) significantly lowered the risk for cardiovascular disease. NCEP ATP I established clear lipid-treatment guidelines to reduce the risk of atherosclerosis.

The importance of this 1984 NCEP ATP I report cannot be overstated: it got the bandwagon rolling to emphasize the importance of lowering lipids to reduce cardiovascular disease.

Largely as a result of the NCEP and AHA cholesterol awareness programs, between 1983 and 1995, the percentage of Americans who had ever had their cholesterol level checked rose from 35% to 75%, an increase of nearly 75 million people. The Third National Health and Nutrition Examination Survey (NHANES III) (1988–1994) showed that since 1978 average total cholesterol levels dropped from 213 to 203, and the prevalence of people with a total cholesterol over 240 fell from 26% to 19%.

Under the guidance of the NIH, these guidelines were revised twice, most recently in 2003 with an update in 2004. All of these shared important similarities: identification of risk classes, the importance of targeting the treatment to the patient's risk, recognition of both HDL and lifestyle, and ever-lower LDL targets. Based on the Treat to New Targets study, the 2004 Update targeted an LDL below 70 for those at very high risk of disease, including secondary prevention and those like diabetics who smoke.

And then in 2013, the NIH exited the guideline writing and turned the process over to the American Heart Association and the American College of Cardiology. The writing committee based its recommendations on a strict interpretation of the literature: namely, the published literature looked at the impact of pre-determined drug doses on lipids and outcomes and did not look at whether an LDL of 60 gave better results than an LDL of 90. (Yes it turns out that atorvastatin 80 gives both a lower LDL and fewer events than atorvastatin 10.) They concluded that the published literature only demonstrated that the benefit lay with the higher dose of the high-intensity statin, but not with the level of LDL achieved.

So now lipid guidelines are both multiple and inconsistent. Internationally there are more than a dozen guidelines and risk calculators. In America alone, there are at least three as of this writing (2013 ACC/AHA, NLA, and AACE). Most guidelines focus on risk assessment and give specific LDL goals. However, the 2013 ACC/AHA guideline primarily assigns the benefit of the treatment to the dose and intensity of the statin based on the patient's risk using the Pooled Cohort Risk Calculator. They did not set LDL targets.

Over the past three years, thinking has continued to evolve. Current thinking (and likely the basis for consideration in future guideline writing) is 1) a continuation of risk assessment tool and risk stratification with 2) treatment correlated with the patient's risk, 3) a return to LDL targets and 4) the addition of non-HDL targets (non-HDL target = LDL target + 30).

The 2013 AHA/ACC Guidelines again (see table 17 below) based their treatment according to the patient's risk of disease. They emphasized the importance of a heart-healthy lifestyle. And they were mute on topics where the literature was not conclusive.

The Pooled Cohort Ten-Year Risk Calculator can be criticized, but is an excellent starting point for risk assessment. It gives both a ten-year and lifetime risk assessment—in young females, the lifetime risk may be more indicative of their risk than their ten-year score. Unfortunately, the Pooled Cohort Ten-year Risk Calculator does not take either family history or hsCRP into consideration.

Table 17 Summary of 2013 ACC/AHA Guidelines

Risk Group	Treatment
High risk 1. All patients > age 21 with LDL 70 to 189 with CVD 2. All patients > age 21 with LDL > 190 3. Diabetics age 40 to 75 with LDL 70 to 189 and who have other risk factors (e.g., smoking)	High-intensity statins to reduce LDL > 50% ▸ Atorva 40 or 80 ▸ Rosuva 20 or 40
Moderate risk 1. Patients age 40 to 75 with diabetes and LDL 70 to 189 and no other risk factors 2. Patients age 40 to 75 without CVD and LDL 70 to 189 and a 10-yr risk > 7.5% using the Pooled Cohort Risk Calculator	Moderate-intensity statin to reduce LDL 30% to 50% CHECK ▸ Atorva 10 to 20 ▸ Fluva 40 bid ▸ Lova 40 ▸ Pitava 2 to 4 ▸ Prava 40 ▸ Rosuva 10 ▸ Simva 20 to 40
Primary prevention 1. Primary prevention patients with risk < 7.5% using the Pooled Cohort Risk Calculator	Use clinical judgment and other factors including ▸ family history, ▸ LDL > 160, ▸ CAC scan > 75th percentile for age, sex, and race, ▸ hsCRP, ▸ ABI < 0.9, or ▸ high lifetime risk

The strongest factor in their regression analysis is increasing age—up to age 75, because beyond that there is no guidance given. The calculator shows that even with optimal CV profiles, the following groups have a risk > 7.5% and need moderate-intensity statins:

- White males > age 62
- White females > age 70
- Black males > age 65
- Black females > age 69

Coronary calcium scans

The 2013 ACC/AHA guidelines mention the use of other non-invasive tests (e.g., coronary calcium scans, ABI, hsCRP) when the individual risk assessment is uncertain. They note that treatment with a moderate-intensity statin is indicated when the CAC score is > 75th percentile for age, sex, and race or > 300. Because the CAC scan and score continue to show superiority in reclassification and ability to predict events but are confusing to some practitioners, we wish to take a few pages to explain the CAC scan and score.

Increasingly, the coronary artery calcium CAC scan is recognized as a superior tool to visualize the extent of coronary atherosclerosis rather than estimate its existence and severity from a calculator. The scan is inexpensive, fast, and low radiation (equivalent to about one and a half mammograms). It is almost never covered by insurance, but often costs only $100.

The report score will be a number. Each pixel with the same density as bone in the distribution of the coronary arteries gets one point. The CAC scan report will give both an absolute score and then where that score places the patient stated as a percentile for age and sex and race.

CAC scans are indicated for patients with a Pooled Cohort Ten-Year Risk between 5% and 7.4%, or when indicated by a strong family history of premature disease in first-degree relatives.

The scan is commonly performed to re-classify the ten-year risk in patients because significant heterogeneity exists in people who otherwise qualify for statins. About half of the patients will have a CAC score of zero and will be reclassified away from statin use. We use the calculator from the Multi-Ethnic Study of Atherosclerosis (Google MESA CAC).

Below we offer two examples showing when the CAC scan was helpful:

- A 48-year-old athletic female nonsmoker with an excellent diet comes to see you because her 52-year-old brother just had an MI and CABG. Her lipid profile shows a TC 217 Trigs 75 HDL 62 LDL 140. Her Pooled Cohort Risk is less than 1%, but family history was not included. Her coronary calcium score was 54, or the 98th percentile.

She was above the 75th percentile for age and sex, and ACC/AHA guidelines say we should treat her. We did.

- A 63-year-old male with pretreatment TC 295, Trigs 150, HDL 50 and LDL 205 and BP 125/84. His ten-year risk by the Pooled Cohort Risk Calculator is 10.4%. He has tried and failed five different statins in varying doses because of severe myalgias and proximal leg weakness. He has developed myalgias from ezetimibe and cannot tolerate bile acid sequestrants. His coronary calcium score was 1. The MESA (Multi-Ethnic Study of Atherosclerosis) 10-year risk calculator with coronary calcium gives him a 2.8% ten-year risk of an event. This is below the threshold of 7.5% for starting a statin. We elected to treat him with lifestyle only and repeat the coronary calcium scan in three years.

The Multi-Ethnic Study of Atherosclerosis calculator has three calculators based on CAC scores. (google MESA CAC). The first is a comprehensive risk calculator incorporating family history and CAC scores. The ten-year risk percentages are given with and without the CAC scores. This allows for an easy reclassification, either up or down, and greater clarity on decision-making discussion. The second calculator on the website gives the CAC score as a percentage based on age, sex, and race. This is important, because most guidelines say to treat if the risk is above the 75th percentile for age, sex, and race. The third calculator converts the CAC score into an estimated arterial age and gives the estimated ten-year risk based on Framingham and the CAC score.

CAC scans are not indicated for high-risk patients. If the patient has a score over 300, the criteria for high risk, the scan need not be repeated.

The 2013 ACC/AHA guidelines indicate that treatment should be implemented for patients who are above the 75th percentile or when the score is over 300. The table below shows that we are far more often dealing with patients with scores over the 75th percentile.

Table 18 75th percentile CAC Scores by age From MESA calculator

	45	50	55	60	65	70	75
White males	0	22	68	155	307	540	820
Black males	0	2	15	40	95	191	331
White females	0	0	1	16	54	119	237
Black females	0	0	0	5	26	77	138

Guidelines from the National Lipid Association

In 2015, the National Lipid Association wrote two guidelines for the treatment of Dyslipidemia in Special Populations (dyslipidemia being their comprehensive word to include all lipid disorders). These can be found at their website lipid.org in the guideline section.

These guidelines are somewhat complex in the name of accuracy and best evidence. The complexity is unfortunate because we understand and support the NLA logic and intent.

Step one of the NLA protocol is to follow sequential steps in ASCVD risk assessment. These are

1. Identify patients at very high- or high-risk
   a. Very high
      i. ASCVD
      ii. Diabetes with > 2 other major risk factors (see below)
   b. High risk
      i. Diabetes with 0-1 other major risk factor
      ii. CKD stage 3B or 4
      iii. LDL > 190
2. Count major ASCVD risk factors (see below)
   a. If 0 to 1 and no other major risk indicators of higher risk (these are not defined), assign to low-risk category
   b. If > 3 major ASCVD, assign to high risk

3. If 2 major risk factors, risk scoring should be considered and additional testing may be useful
   a. If score is high risk, assign to high risk
   b. If there is no above indication, assign to moderate risk

Major risk factors for ASCVD according to the NLA guidelines:

1. Age
   a. Males > 45
   b. Females > 50
2. Family history of premature CAD
   a. < 55 if male first-degree relative
   b. < 65 if female first-degree relative
3. Current cigarette smoker
4. BP > 140/90 or on Rx
5. Low HDl
   a. Male < 40
   b. Female < 50

They identify the following as high- or very high-risk groups who do not need further risk assessment and should instead be treated:

1. Diabetes types 1 or 2
2. CKD > stage 3B
3. LDL > 190
4. Known ASCVD (CAD, TIA or ischemic stroke, PAD or ABI < 0.9, documented atherosclerosis)

The NLA guidelines suggests treatment with moderate- to high-intensity statins to an LDL goal for the following risk groups.

Table 19 NLA Guidelines for ASCVD risk assessment and treatment goals

		Consider Rx		Treatment goal	
Risk	Criteria	LDL	Non-HDL	LDL	Non-HDL
Low	▸ 0–1 major factor* ▸ other **	> 160	> 190	< 100	< 130
Moderate	▸ 0-1 major factor ▸ risk scoring ▸ other **	> 130	> 160	< 100	< 130

High	▸ > 3 major factors
	▸ DM (1 &2) and
	  ▸ 0–1 major risk factor
	  ▸ no end organ damage
	▸ CKD 3B or 4
	▸ Risk score in high category
	▸ LDL > 190
		> 100	> 130	< 100	< 130

Very high	▸ ASCVD
	▸ DM (1 or 2) and
	  ▸ > 1 major risk factor
	  ▸ End organ damage
		> 70	> 100	< 70	< 100

* major risk factors = male > 44, female > 54, + FH of early CAD, current smoker, BP > 140/90 or Rx, and HDL < 40 if male and < 50 if female
**other = smoking, family history, CAC > 300, metabolic syndrome, hsCRP > 2, Lp(a) > 50

Unfortunately, the 2015 NLA guidelines assign patients with an LDL > 190 to a footnote in their table 3. It says LDL> L > 190, consider severe hypercholesterolemia phenotype, which includes familial hypercholesterolemia. Lifestyle intervention and pharmacotherapy is recommended for adults with severe hypercholesterolemic phenotype.

Other guidelines

Recently, several major organizations have issued alternative guidelines or consensus panel reports to address these issues. Below, are the (1) treatment guidelines of the Canadian Cardiovascular Society, (2) the American Association of Clinical Endocrinologists' opinion on the lipid targets of patients with pre-diabetes, and (3) the recommendations of the American

Diabetes Association and the American College of Cardiology Foundation on lipid management of patients with metabolic syndrome.

In 2009, the Canadian Cardiovascular Society issued their guidelines for lipid management. They are summarized in the following table.

Table 20 Treatment Lipid Targets from the 2009 Canadian Guidelines
Canadian lab values expressed as mmol/L have been converted to the American mg/dL
Adapted from Genest, J. Can J Cardiol 2009;24:567–579

Risk level	Initiate treatment if:	Primary targets			
		LDL-C	Evidence class/level	Apo B	Evidence class/level
High risk	CAD Most pts with DM FRS > 20%	< 77 or ≥ 50% LDL-C	I/A	< 80	I/A
Moderate FRS 10% to 20%	LDL-C > 135 TC/HDL > 5.0 hs-CRP > 2.0 mg/L Men > 50 Women > 60 FH and hsCRP modulates risk (RRS)	< 77 or ≥ 50% LDL-C	IIa/A	< 80	II/A
Low risk FRS < 10%	LDL-C ≥ 193	≥ 50% LDL-C	IIa/A		

Once the LDL-C and apo B are at goal, the Canadian Guidelines have optional secondary targets for (1) an TC:HDL-C < 4.0; (2) a non-HDL-C < 140; (3) triglycerides < 150; (4) apo B: apo A1 < 0.8; and (5) hsCRP < 2.0.

In 2008, the American Association of Clinical Endocrinologists (Garber AJ et al. Endo Pact 14; 7: 933–946) wrote a position paper looking at when the risks of diabetes really start. They concluded that patients with prediabetes should be treated to the same risk factor targets as patients with diabetes.

In 2008, the American Diabetes Association and the American College of Cardiology Foundation published a consensus statement with more guidance for treating these at-risk patients with metabolic syndrome (Brunzell et al. Diabetes Care (2008) 31; 4: 811–819). They define a very high-risk group as those with (1) known CVD or those (2) who do not yet have CVD but do have diabetes and one or more cardiometabolic risk factors beyond their dyslipidemia. The recommended treatment goals for this group are (1) LDL-C < 70, (2) non-HDL-C < 100, and (3) apo B < 80. They define a high-risk group as (1) those without diabetes or clinical CVD but with two or more major CVD risk factors such as smoking, hypertension, and family history of premature CVD or (2) those with diabetes but no other CVD risk factors. The recommended treatment goals for this group are (1) LDL-C < 100, (2) non-HDL-C < 130, and (3) apo B < 90.

Table 21 Criteria and treatment goals for patients with cardiometabolic risk based on the consensus statement of the American Diabetes Association and the American College of Cardiology Foundation

Adapted from Brunzell et al. Diabetes Care (2008) 31; 4: 811–819

Group	Definitions	Goals
Highest risk	Known CVD or Patients who do not yet have CVD but do have diabetes and one or more cardiometabolic risk factors beyond their dyslipidemia	LDL-C < 70 non-HDL-C < 100 and apo B < 80
High-risk	Patients without diabetes or clinical CVD but with two or more major CVD risk factors such as smoking, hypertension, and family history of premature CVD or Patients with diabetes but no other CVD risk factors	LDL-C < 100 non-HDL-C < 130 and apo B < 90

Chapter 9
LIPID MEDICATIONS

LIPID-LOWERING MEDICATIONS OFFER the best method to reduce the burden of premature atherosclerosis, cardiovascular disease, and mortality. Four medications (statins, intestinal cholesterol absorption blockers, the bile acid sequestrants, and the PCSK9 inhibitors) primarily lower plasma LDL-C, LDL-P, and apo B. Three medications (niacin, fibrates, and omega-3 oils) primarily lower triglycerides while niacin, and to a lesser degree, fibrates also raise HDL-C. Each of these six medication classes also impacts all other lipid lines, and they are often combined to maximize their benefit. This chapter will discuss each of the drugs separately. The following chapter will discuss how the drugs are best used in various clinical settings and combinations.

This chapter will discuss lipid-altering medications in the following order.

1. Statins
2. Bile acid sequestrants
3. Intestinal absorption inhibitors
4. PCSK9 inhibitors
5. Niacin
6. Fibrates
7. Omega-3 fatty acids

Effects of lipid-lowering medications

Each of the six classes of lipid-altering medications has a specific lipid target but also impacts other lipid parameters. These effects are summarized in Table 14. For example, depending on the statin and the dose selected, you can expect that statins will lower LDL-C by 20% to 65%, lower TG by 10% to 35%, raise HDL-C by 5% to 15%, lower both Lp-PLA2 and CRP, but not affect the level of Lp(a).

Table 22 Effect of lipid-lowering drugs in percentage

	LDL-C	TG	HDL-C	Lp(a)
Primary LDL-C lowering medications				
Statins	↓ 20 – 65	↓ 10 – 35*	↑ 5 – 15	0
Ezetimibe	↓ 20	0	0	0
Bile acid sequestrants	↓ 15 – 30	↑ to ↑↑ if TG > 400 at start	↑ 5	0
PCSK9 inhibitors	↓ 50%			↓ 25%
Primary triglyceride lowering medications				
Fibrates	0 to ↓ 10 May ↑ if TG > 400	↓ 30 – 50	↑ 5 – 20	0 to ↓
Niacin	↓ 5 to 25	↓ 20 – 50	↑ 15 – 35	↓
Omega 3	0 but may ↑ if TG > 400	↓ 35 – 50	↑ 5	0
* Will lower TG more if starting TG is > 400				

Medications that primarily lower LDL-C, non-HDL-C, and apo B

The primary purpose of lipid treatment is to lower the risk of cardiovascular disease. Virtually every study has shown that whenever the LDL-C was lowered and regardless of the method (intestinal bypass, bile acid sequestrants, niacin, or statins), the risk of coronary events also declined.

Four medications lower LDL-C: the statins, bile acid sequestrants, the intestinal cholesterol absorption blockers, and the new PCSK9 inhibitors.

The Statins

We devote a considerable chunk of this text to statins because well over 20 million American adults currently take a statin.

Statins are a potent LDL-C-lowering drug class, and one of our most powerful tools to reduce the risk of cardiovascular disease. Statins are the only lipid-altering class of drugs that demonstrate clear improvements in mortality in both primary and secondary prevention. For every mmol or roughly 40 mg of LDL lowering, statins lower major adverse cardiac events and cardiac death by 25% to 30%. They are effective in both men and women regardless of age (although relatively little data in those > age 75), regardless of the starting LDL, in primary and secondary prevention, type 1 and type 2 diabetics, regardless of blood pressure or BMI, in all ethnic populations, and all underlying disease states with the exception of end-stage renal disease patients on dialysis.

All of the available science shows that lowering LDL reduces CVD, and the lower the LDL, the greater the benefit. But the science also shows that atherosclerosis is caused by the apo B lipoproteins and not by the LDL-C. In other words, to really maximally lower the risk of CVD, our treatments should lower apo B and non-HDL-C to the same population percentiles as LDL-C. This becomes problematic because statins lower LDL-C an average of 42%, non-HDL-C 39%, and apo B by 33%. (Sniderman, AD *Journal of Clin Lipid* (2008) 2: 36–42) This means that treating LDL-C to goal often leaves an apo B that is substantially above goal. In other words, to be maximally effective, we need to get non-HDL-C and apo B to goal, which often requires higher doses, higher potency statins, or combination therapies.

Table 15 below lists major placebo-controlled, randomized, double-blind trials with statins. The patients in these trials included those with and without known CAD, smokers and non-smokers, the young and the old, diabetics and non-diabetics, and people with both abnormal and "normal" lipids. The studies total an impressive 422,000 person-years. The conclusion is quite clear: statins lower LDL-C effectively and they substantially lower coronary events and deaths.

Please keep in mind that this statin-induced 30% reduction in coronary events and death is wonderful, but still leaves 70% of the cardiovascular risk. This so-called "residual risk" is the new target of even lower LDL-C targets and combination therapies.

Table 23 The impact of major statin trials covering 422,000 person-years of data in placebo-controlled, randomized, double-blind clinical-event endpoint trials (adapted from Ballytine p. 265)

Trial	Statin	Change in LDL-C in %	Change in coronary deaths or non-fatal MI in %
4S	Simva 40	−35	−34
LIPID	Prava 40	−25	−24
CARE	Prava 40	−32	−24
HPS	Simva 40	−32	−27
ALERT	Fluva 40	−32	−35
ALLHAT-LLT	Prava 40	−17	−9
PROSPER	Prava 40	−27	−19
ASCOT-LLA	Atorva 10	−35	−36
LIPS	Fluva 80	−27	−31
SPARCL	Atorva 80	−45	−35
CARDS	Atorva 10	−31	−35
WOSCOPS	Prava 40	−26	−31
AFCAPS/TexCAPS	Lova 20–40	−25	−40
Average		**−29.9**	**−29.2**

A 2013 Cochrane Review of 18 randomized control trials covering 56,000 patients showed that statins lowered mortality 14%, CHD by 27%, stroke by 22%, nonfatal MI by 33%, and revascularization by 38%. It is awfully hard to argue that statins don't work, or that their side effects are worse than their benefits. The evidence to the positive is overwhelming.

Mechanism

All statins work in the liver. They block the hepatic production of cholesterol, which the liver needs for the production of bile. Sensing a shortage of cholesterol, the liver up-regulates its LDL-Receptors to pull cholesterol from the systemic circulation. This up-regulation lowers the circulating LDL-P, LDL-C, IDL-P, and VLDL-P. The majority of LDL-C lowering is caused by this up-regulation of hepatic LDL-R, but statins have some additional LDL-C lowering effects because they cause a smaller hepatic pool of cholesterol. Statins also—and counterintuitively—upregulate PCSK9.

Following is the same explanation slightly more detailed. Statins competitively inhibit the enzyme 3-hydroxy-3-methylglutaryl-coenzyme A (HMG-CoA), which is the ratelimiting step in the intra-hepatocyte formation of cholesterol. This decreases the intra-hepatic cholesterol pool, which upregulates the nuclear-transcription factors (called sterolregulatory-element binding proteins, SREBPs) to increase the number of surface LDL-R. These LDL-R bind with and remove the circulating apo B and apo E lipoproteins (LDL-P, VLDL-P, and IDL-P) to replenish the hepatic cholesterol pool. The up-regulation of LDL-R also lowers triglyceride levels because LDL-R also binds with the triglyceride-rich VLDL-P and IDL-P.

Other effects and therapeutic uses of the statins

Statins reliably lower LDL-C by 20% to 65%, lower triglycerides by 10% to 35%, and raise HDL by 5% to 15%. The triglyceride-lowering effect of statins is proportional to the starting triglyceride level. However, statins do lower elevated triglycerides quite well, and three statins (atorva, simva, and rosuva) have an FDA indication for hypertriglyceridemia.

In addition to improving the lipid profile and independent of their effect on LDL-C, statins have other pleotropic effects that help to reduce cardiovascular disease. Statins are anti-inflammatory by lowering hsCRP and Lp-PLA-2, stabilize plaques by inhibiting vascular metalloproteinases, are antithrombotic, and promote nitric oxide production to enhance endothelial function. All of these pleotrophic effects contribute to statin's ability to lower cardiovascular disease and mortality.

In February 2010, the US Food and Drug Administration (FDA) approved rosuvastatin to reduce the risk of a CVD event in men ≥ 50 and women ≥ 60 with an hsCRP ≥ 2 and the presence of at least one additional CVD risk factor, such as hypertension, low HDL-C, smoking, or a family history. This recommendation was based on the JUPITER study, where rosuva 20 reduced the relative risk a CVD event by 50% compared to a placebo. Note that rosuva was not effective in people with an elevated CRP and no other CV risk factor.

Because the absolute risk is highest, statins have the lowest number-needed-to-treat in patients who already have occlusive vascular disease; elevated LDL-C, hypertriglyceridemia, or evidence of inflammation; are diabetics; or have either severe or multiple risk factors for cardiovascular disease. However, statins may actually be most beneficial when used appropriately in primary prevention where they effectively reduce and delay the onset of major cardiovascular events. In the primary prevention setting the risk-to-benefit ratio must be considered, which is why statins are recommended when the ten-year risk exceeds 7.5%.

The various statins

Today, there are seven statins on the market: atorva, fluva, lova, pitava, prava, simva, and rosuva. An eighth statin, cerivastatin, was on the market briefly, but was removed because it was associated with a very high incidence of rhabdomyolysis, particularly when combined with gemfibrozil. Much of the public fear about statin use lingers from these well-publicized complications of a now-discontinued drug.

Chart 3 Power of each statin by dose to lower LDL-C
(Adapted and modified from the National Lipid Association Self-Assessment Program, Basic Lipid and Lipoprotein Metabolism, Diagnosis and Treatment of Dyslipidemia, Critique Book, Aug 2008, p 22)

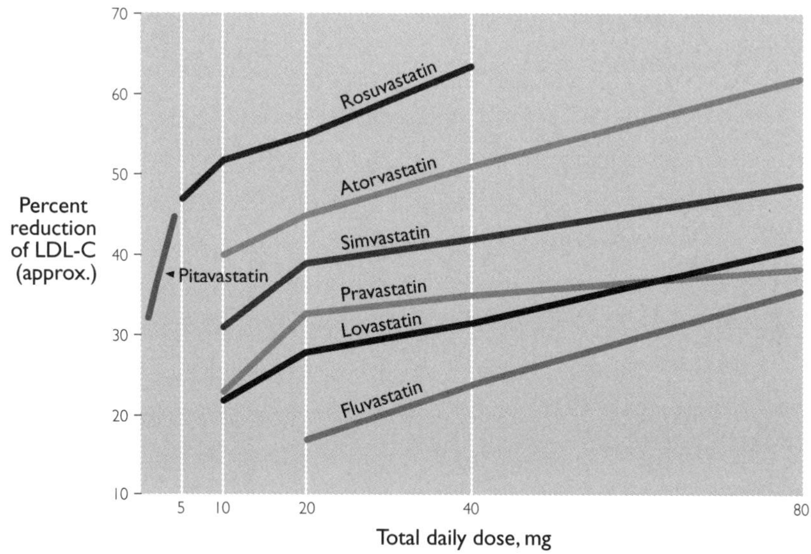

The different statins each reduce LDL-C to a different extent. A 20 mg tablet of fluva might lower LDL-C by 20%, while a 1 mg of pitava can lower LDL-C by 32%, and 10 mg rosuva can lower LDL-C by more than 50%. This is an important but often misunderstood concept. The 2013 ACC/AHA Guidelines identified moderate- and high-intensity statins and used them respectively for moderate- to high-risk patients. The moderate-intensity statins are those that lower LDL 30% to 50%, and the high-intensity statins lower LDL more than 50%. The high-intensity statins are atorva 40 and 80 and rosuva 20 and 40. The list moderate-intensity statins are listed in table 23 below.

All guidelines base the decision to treat on the patient's risk. But once the decision has been made to treat the patient, then the LDL should be lowered by at least 30%. This is an important concept because it is not appropriate to initiate treatment of a high-risk patient with a low- or moderate-intensity statin like prava 40 or simva 10.

Table 24 Statin doses by intensity in mg

	Doses for high intensity to lower LDL-C by > 50%	Doses for moderate intensity to lower LDL-C by 30% to 50%	Doses for low intensity to lower LDL-C by < 30%
Atorva	40 or 80	10 or 20	5
Fluva		80	20
Lova		40	20
Pitava		2 or 4	1
Prava		40 or 80	10 or 20
Rosuva	20 or 40	5 or 10	2.5
Simva		20 or 40	10

Special notes on statins

Statins have many quirks, both as a class and individually.

- Many Asians are sensitive to statins, necessitating a (much) lower-than-normal starting dose. The dose can be adjusted upward if necessary at the later visit.
- Some people have genetic mutations that reduce the metabolism of statins. These people are likely to be unable to tolerate statins and need non-statin therapies.
- The half-life of statins varies considerably. Atorva, pitava, and rosuva have a half-life of 20+ hours, so they can be taken any time of day or in alternate-day dosing. The remaining statins have a half-life of about six hours and need to be taken in the evening, because most hepatic cholesterol synthesis takes place at night.
- Lova is best absorbed if taken with food.

- Many statins have potentially important drug or disease interactions that limit either the use or dosing strength.
- Statins should be continued during hospitalization. There is some evidence for a rebound endothelial and inflammatory reaction when statins are stopped abruptly.

Adverse drug interactions of the statins

In this section, we will discuss statin side effects and interactions with other medications.

Statin side effects

Statins have several minor side effects, a few moderate side effects (enough to stop the medication) and rare real side effects, all of which are grossly exaggerated by television media stars and the internet charlatans. To them, statins are the devil in pill form. To the authors and all scientific experts, statins are among the safest and most effective medications.

In fact, statins are among the safest pills that your patients will take. Which is safer: statins or acetaminophen or aspirin? Clearly statins. Your hospital admits patients every year for liver disease due to unintentional acetaminophen overdose, and acetaminophen overdose is a common method of suicide. Do they ever admit anyone for statin overdose? Aspirin and bleeding are a common reason for admission and complications. Statins and complications severe enough to require admission? Very rare, and likely rhabdomyolysis when it happens.

We will address the side effects seen with statins and muscles, statins and diabetes, statins and memory issues.

Statin myalgias are real and occur in 5% to 7% of patients. Fortunately, they are not nearly as severe as the internet anti-statin web sites would have our patients believe. Many patients starting a statin will notice some mild muscle ache or an extra charley horse for a week or two. Some people have ongoing aches or arthralgias but not severe enough to stop the medication. A small percentage of patients will have enough muscle pain that they stop the statin.

When patients stop statins, we do the following:

1. Check for drug-drug interactions. We have had patients on stable doses of atorva develop rhabdomyolysis when a CYP450 medication like erythromycin or amiodarone was started.
2. Check vitamin D and TSH levels. If low, either can increase risk of myalgias. Replace as necessary and restart a different statin at a lower dose.
3. Change to a lower-dose of a statin with a different metabolism. For example, if the patient gets myalgias on atorvastatin, you might switch to rosuvastatin or pravastatin. And / or switch to a much lower dose of rosuvastatin like 2.5 mg three days a week (e.g., Monday, Wednesday, and Friday) and then increase as tolerated or add ezetimibe. In our experience we can often achieve 40% LDL reductions with this later method.
4. Some patients tolerate statins for weeks or months and then develop the myalgias. The myalgias will resolve once the statin is stopped. We often have these patients take a two-week drug holiday and then restart the same statin.
5. Fluva, pitava, and prava are often surprisingly well tolerated in patients with myalgias. These should be tried before you declare total statin intolerance.

Rarely statins unmask an underlying muscle disease. These patients have severe myalgias and weakness, usually proximal. The authors take weakness seriously and immediately stop the statin. You need to check the CK to exclude rhabdomyolysis, but a normal CK does not preclude serious statin muscle injury. These patients should be referred to a lipidologist and perhaps a neuromuscular specialists if the weakness persists or is severe, because they may have carnitine palmitoyltransferase (CPT) deficiency.

Statins have been associated with an increased risk of diabetes. In the studies, diabetes more commonly developed in people who had prediabetes or were obese than the people without risk factors for diabetes.

In the JUPITER trial, the benefit of statins outweighed the risk of developing diabetes. In patients with no diabetes risk factors (6,095 people), there was a 52% reduction (N = 86) in vascular events or deaths in the statin treatment arm and no new diabetes. In the 11,500 patients with a risk factor for diabetes, 134 vascular events or deaths were avoided at the cost of 54 new cases of diabetes. (Ridker et al, Lancet 2012).

Statin labels also now contain a warning about possible memory loss or confusion. These are rare side effects that resolve when the statin is stopped.

Statins were once thought to increase liver enzymes, but liver damage from statins is rare. The FDA now recommends that liver enzymes be tested before starting the statin (to exclude active hepatitis where statins are contraindicated) but no longer recommends ongoing or routine liver enzyme testing.

Statins have a host of drug-drug interactions. We will discuss them first as interactions with other lipid medications, then as drugs that compete for P450 enzyme CYP3A4 metabolism, and then as drugs that decrease statin levels. These are summarized in Table 17.

Statin interactions with other lipid medications

Statins are often used with other lipid-lowering medications, sometimes with three or more lipid-lowering medications. These combinations are associated with increased risks, most notably myopathies or elevated liver enzymes.

Statins and fibrates

Statins are often used in combination with fibrates, particularly in patients with elevated triglycerides as often seen with insulin resistance.

Statins and fibrates can cause myalgias, myopathies, and rhabdomyolysis. The statin-fibrate interaction is far more likely to occur when statins are used with gemfibrozil than when statins are used with fenofibrate or fenofibric acid. The 2009 Canadian Guidelines actually recommend against using gemfibrozil with statins because of the problems with rhabdomyolysis. Gemfibrozil and statins both compete for the glucuronidation process. This competition increases the serum concentration of statins which increases the risk of myopathies including rhabdomyolysis. This competition for the glucuronidation metabolism process applies to all statins, but was most marked when gemfibrozil was used with cerivastatin, which has been withdrawn from the market for this reason. If you must use gemfibrozil (usually because the patient has renal disease or formulary limitations), you should consider limiting your statin to atorva or fluva, which seem to have fewer problems when taken with gemfibrozil.

Chart 4 Rhabdomyolysis occurs 15 times more frequently when statins are combined with gemfibrozil than when statins are used with fenofibrates.
(Jones, Am J Cardiol. 2005; 95: 120–122)

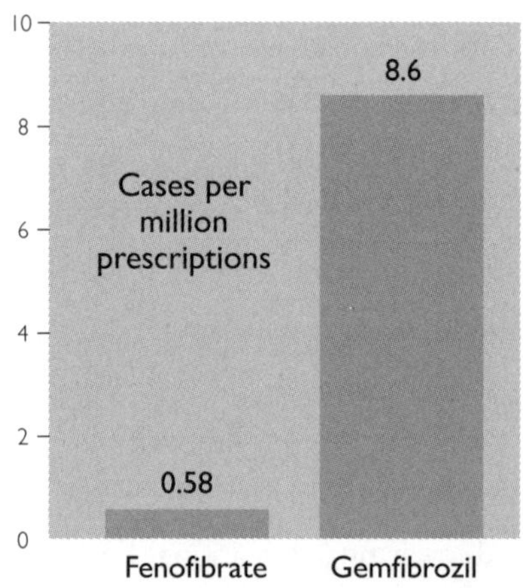

The risk of myopathy is also reduced if, when the patient is on gemfibrozil, you limit the statin to no more than a moderate dose. Gemfibrozil doubles the C_{max} of lova, prava, rosuva, and simva, while other fenofibrates do not appreciably affect the C_{max} of statins. (Bellosa, *Circ* 2004; 109 (suppl III): 50–57)

Fenofibrates and fenofibric acid do not have this competition for glucuronidation and are much safer to use with statins. The product information on fenofibric acid does not contain special cautionary language on use with statins, but does note that rhabdomyolysis has occurred in patients on fenofibric acid.

Statins and niacin

Niacin may exacerbate the hepatic effects of some statins. The slow-release niacin, which have minimal flushing, are metabolized by the low-capacity system in the liver. The immediate-release niacin (Niacor) and extended-release niacin (Niaspan) are metabolized by the higher capacity system in the liver and associated with more flushing. (See the niacin section on page 92.) Liver enzymes should be checked in patients who are on both a statin and a niacin.

Statin interactions with other lipid-lowering medications

Statins have minimal drug interactions if given with ezetimibe or bile acid sequestrants, because these two drugs stay primarily within the gut. However, in rare patients and though a not-yet-understood pathway, the combination of ezetimibe and a statin can increase liver enzymes or cause myositis.

Statin interactions with other medications

Statins are metabolized by CYP3A4 or CYP2C9 or have minimal CYP450 metabolism. Table 17 summarizes the important statin-drug interactions and recommended maximum dose of statins. There is no need to memorize this unless you are taking the lipid boards; just know that it is here and refer to it when necessary, or ask your clinic pharmacist for help getting the most current information.

The statin-drug interaction chart groups all of the CYP3A4 medications together, because they more often have drug interactions with the statins.

Table 25 Statin-drug interaction with some common medications

Categories: Contra-indicated means contra-indicated

Avoid means avoid unless the potential benefit outweighs the potential risk

Dose indication means max dose recommended and close monitoring required

Monitor means extra awareness and monitoring required

OK means that only routine awareness and monitoring are appropriate (i.e., no special drug-drug interaction was noted in the reference source)

Reference is both package inserts and Micromedex2.0 by Thompson Reuters accessed online Aug 31,2010 http://www.thomsonhc.com/hcs/librarian/PFPUI/qN1iF7z1wxHDXC

Always check most current drug-drug interaction charts before prescribing

	CYP450 3A4			CYP450 2C9	Minimal CYP450		
	Atorva	**Lova**	**Simva**	**Fluva**	**Prava**	**Pitava**	**Rosuva**
Fenofibric acid	OK	OK	OK	OK	OK	OK	OK
Gemfibrozil	Monitor	20 max	10 max	Avoid	Monitor	Monitor	10 max
Niacin	Monitor	20 max	Monitor	Monitor	Monitor	Monitor	Monitor
Ezetimibe	OK	OK	OK	OK	OK	OK	OK
Diltiazem	Monitor	20 max	10 max	OK	OK	OK	OK
Verapamil	Monitor	20 max	10 max	OK	OK	OK	OK
Amiodarone	Monitor	40 max	20 max	OK	OK	OK	Monitor
Erythromycin	Avoid	Hold statin during erythro-mycin Rx	Hold statin during erythro-mycin Rx	Monitor	Avoid	1 max	OK
Azithromycin	Monitor	Monitor	Monitor	OK	OK	OK	OK
Cyclosporine	Contra-indicated	Contra-indicated	Contra-indicated	20 max (may be best statin)	20 max	Contra-indicated	5 max

Grapefruit juice may also raise the AUC of atorva, lova, and simva. It is probably best to limit grapefruit juice to a regular glass (e.g., avoid large quantities, and by that we mean more than a pint a day).

Medications and supplements that decrease the effectiveness of some statins

Other medications and herbals induce CYP3A4, and these decrease the effectiveness particularly of the CYP3A4-metabolized statins (atorva, lova, and simva). These include (alphabetically)

- barbiturates
- carbamazepine
- dexmethasone
- glucocorticoids
- modafinal
- nevaripine
- phenobarbital
- phenylbutazone
- phenytoin
- St. Johns Wort
- rifampin
- sulfinpyrazone

Potential muscle problems with statins

Statins cause muscle problems in some patients. When these occur, patients most often have myalgias; only rarely do they have myopathy, and even more rarely rhabdomyolysis.

First, let's define the terms so we are all talking the same language.

- Myalgias are muscle aches with no CK increase
- Myopathy is defined as muscle aches with a CK > 10 times normal
- Rhabdomyolysis is muscle aches with a CK > 10 and an elevated creatinine

Myalgias occur in 2% to 11% of patients taking statins, a rate similar to that observed in placebo groups. A meta-analysis of 21 randomized, placebo-controlled trials with 180,000 person-years of data showed that myopathy occurred in 5 patients per 100,000 person-years and rhabdomyolysis occurred in 3.4 per 100,000 person-years. An in-depth study of the statin safety in the AERS database found 0.3 to 2.2 cases of myopathy and 0.3 to 13.5 cases of rhabdomyolysis per one million statin prescriptions. (Law and Rudnicka *Am J Cardiol* 2006; 97: S52–S60)

Table 26 Incident rates of rhabdomyolysis from a managed care claims database of 875,000 statin users (Cziraky et al. *Am J Cardiol* 2006; 97(supp): 61C–68C)

	Rate per 100,000 person years
Atrova	6
Fluva	16
Lova	3
Prava	11
Simva	6
Rosuva	12
Ceriva—WITHDRAWN	84

There are also dose-related differences in the likelihood of a statin-caused myopathy (weakness or myalgias plus CK > 10 times normal). For all statins, the higher the dose, the greater the likelihood of myopathy. Some experts even say that the risk of myopathy varies by a factor of 10 from lowest to highest dose. The combination of a lower-dose statin plus ezetimibe avoids this risk of myalgia and myopathy. Adding ezetimibe to a statin has the same LDL-C lowering effect as increasing the statin from the lowest to the highest dose.

Statin-related muscle complications are more common (1) with highest doses of any statin; or (2) in a patient who is elderly, has a small body size, renal dysfunction, obstructive hepatic disease, hypothyroidism, or poly-pharmacy.

The risk of myopathy is lowest with prava, which has no cases of serious myopathy in 112,000 person-years of data collected. Prava, fluva, and rosuva are hydrophilic and, in theory, should penetrate the muscle less than the hydrophobic statins. However, some patients are sensitive to all statins and others will find one statin that works without causing myalgias. Alternatives for patients with statin-related myalgias are shown in Chapter 9, Strategy 6 on page 140.

Symptoms of myopathy may occur at any time during treatment, but are most common within the first few months. Whenever the CK rises > 10 times normal, the statin should be stopped. The CK elevation will resolve within one month in half the patients, and within 6 months in the remainder. These patients do not require any other therapy for their elevated CK.

National Lipid Association Recommendations for Statin-Related Muscle Issues

The National Lipid Association makes the following recommendations for management of muscle symptoms:

Baseline CK testing

Obtain baseline CK only in high-risk patients, those with renal or liver disease, poly-pharmacy, or underlying and predisposing disease. CK testing is optional for others.

Routine CK testing

CK measurements in asymptomatic patients are not recommended. (You run the risk of finding a borderline elevated CK in an asymptomatic patient and then inappropriately stopping the statin.)

If muscle symptoms occur

Measure CK if muscle symptoms occur

Exclude other causes of myalgia such as falls, seizures, hypothyroidism, increased physical activity, and ask about large quantities (> 8 ounces) of grapefruit juice, herbs, or any other medications that might interfere with statin metabolism.

If intolerable muscle symptoms occur

Stop the statin and, after the patient becomes asymptomatic, consider restarting at a lower dose or different statin (see Strategy 6 in Chapter 9 for tricks to successfully re-start statins or other alternatives in patients with intolerable myopathy).

Muscle symptoms and CK elevated

< 10 times normal	Continue the statin and monitor
≥ 10 times normal	Stop statin

CK and creatinine both elevated

Stop statin, consider rhabdomyolysis

Potential liver problems with the statins

The ability of statins to cause liver damage has been exaggerated. Statins increase liver enzymes over 3 times normal only slightly more commonly than placebo and they cause liver failure at the same rate of the general population not on statins. As with CK elevation, there is a direct correlation between the minimum and maximum dose of the statin's propensity to increase LFTs. And LFTs are more likely to increase when other medications with hepatic metabolism are combined.

Statins may be given safely to patients with mild liver enzyme elevation such as nonalcoholic fatty liver disease. Statins may be part of a therapeutic regimen (lifestyle) for patients with mild liver enzyme elevation due to the atherogenic dyslipidemia of the metabolic syndrome, because they help to lower the triglycerides.

National Lipid Association Recommendations for statins and liver enzymes

The National Lipid Association makes the following recommendations for management of liver enzymes and statins:

Baseline LFT testing

Liver enzymes should be measured before starting statins. Elevations should be investigated before the statin is started. Statins may be used safely in cases of NASH, where obesity or insulin resistance is the likely cause of the elevated LFTs.

Routine LFT testing

Routine LFT measurements are not indicated.

If LFTs elevated 1 to 3 times normal

The statin may be continued safely. The LFTs should be repeated. If the LFTs are still elevated 1 X to 3 X normal, the physician should consider other causes, and use clinical judgment to decide whether to continue the statin, reduce its dose, or discontinue it until the LFT situation has resolved.

If liver damage is suspected or LFTs elevated > 3 times normal

Hepatomegaly, jaundice, and elevated bilirubin are far better indicators of liver damage than isolated LFT elevations. If these are present for whatever reason, the statin should be discontinued. A referral to a gastroenterologist is recommended.

Statins are the mainstay of LDL-C lowering therapy, a therapy proven to lower the risk of cardiovascular events and mortality. We need to continue to keep the problems associated with statins in perspective: when all is said and done, statins substantially reduce the risk of cardiovascular morbidity and death caused by atherosclerosis.

Bile Acid Sequestrants

Bile acid sequestrants, including both resins and polymers, lower LDL-C by binding with bile acids in the gut. Interestingly, while they lower both plasma LDL-C and the incidence of coronary events by 20%, they have a minimal effect on CV mortality.

Mechanism

Bile acid sequestrants bind with bile acids in the gut (70% of the intra-intestinal cholesterol is biliary and 30% is dietary). This decreases the amount of cholesterol exposed to the ileal bile acid transporter enzyme (IBAT). This, in turn, reduces the enterohepatic recirculation of bile salts, which up-regulates 7-α-hydroxylase, the rate-limiting enzyme for the conversion of cholesterol into bile acids, and this increases the liver's requirement for and uptake of cholesterol from the plasma LDL-R.

Effects and therapeutic uses

Bile acid sequestrants lower LDL-C by 15% to 25%. They may minimally increase the HDL-C. The effect on triglycerides is variable and depends largely on the starting triglyceride level. If the starting triglyceride levels are normal or modestly elevated (to the 300 range), then BAS will have a minimal impact on triglycerides. However, if the starting triglyceride levels are greater than 400, BAS will raise the triglycerides, sometimes substantially. Fasting triglycerides over 500 are a contra-indication to starting bile acid sequestrants.

Colesevelam also has an FDA indication for use in type 2 diabetes.

The various bile acid sequestrants

Forty years ago, bile acid resins were among the first drugs to show a reduction in CV events—of course, they were almost the only lipid altering drugs available at the time.

The available resins include cholestyramine and colestipol. These have frequent GI side effects which reduce patient compliance and impair the absorption of many drugs but are generic.

A new bile acid sequestrant polymer is colesevelam, a water insoluble polymer that is not absorbed systemically. Its unique biochemical polymer structure has better GI tolerability and fewer drug interactions. Colesevelam is not absorbed into systemic circulation making it the only cholesterol-lowering agent that is probably safe to use in pregnancy—officially it is Pregnancy Class B and should only be used in pregnancy if clearly indicated—and then only by a lipid specialist. Colesevelam also has an adjunct indication for glucose control in type 2 diabetes.

Table 27 Bile acid-binding resins

Generic	Trade	Initial dose	Maximum daily dose
Cholestyramine	Questran	4 gm BID	24 gm divided
Colesevelam	Welchol	625 mg tablet	3 tabs BID
Colestipol	Colestid	5 gm bid	30 gm divided

Side effects

The early drugs cholestyramine and colestipol caused substantial gastrointestinal problems. The newer bile absorption resin colesevelam has fewer GI side effects. Nonetheless, the same precautions apply to all drugs in this class.

BAS causes constipation, bloating, and gas, often bothersome enough to limit patient compliance. BAS may also increase the LFTs if used with statins; this requires LFT monitoring. They may also interfere with the absorption of fat soluble vitamins and many medications. BAS should be taken at least one hour after or four hours before other medications.

Contra-indications

Bile acid sequestrants are contra-indicated when the starting triglycerides are over 500, in patients who have had hypertriglyceridemia-induced pancreatitis, and in patients with a history of bowel obstructions.

Special uses

Welchol is probably the safest LDL-C lowering medication for use during pregnancy, but you should always follow the package insert. Officially, it is Pregnancy Class B and should only be used in pregnancy if clearly indicated.

The package insert also lists an indication of improving glycemic control in type 2 diabetics, although not as monotherapy.

Intestinal Sterol Absorption Blockers

The only approved intestinal sterol absorption blocker is ezetimibe. It is a selective blocker of NPC1L1, the enzyme responsible for the absorption of intestinal sterols. Remember that under normal conditions, the non-cholesterol phytosterols are immediately kicked back into the gut by the action of enzymes ABCG-5/8 and never reach systemic circulation.

Ezetimibe is indicated to lower both LDL-C and apo B alone or in combination with a statin or with fenofibrate, and to reduce the phytosterols in patients with homozygous sitosterolemia (phytosterolemia).

Mechanism

By blocking cholesterol uptake by the enzyme NPC1L1, ezetimibe lowers the concentration of cholesterol esters in chylomicrons, which reduces the amount of cholesterol delivered to the liver by the chylomicron. This in turn up-regulates the LDL-R to pull LDL-P and LDL-C from systemic circulation to maintain adequate levels of cholesterol in the liver for bile production.

Ezetimibe blocks nearly 50% of cholesterol absorption from the gut, but only reduces the plasma cholesterol level by about 20%. Note that this 20% is conveniently the same as the effect of tripling the dose of any statin. (Remember doubling the dose of any statin only decreases the serum cholesterol another 6%. For example, adding ezetimibe 10 to atorva 10 lowers LDL-C as much as going all the way from atorva 10 to atorva 80.)

Ezetimibe is recycled through the enterocyte back into the intestine so there is minimal systemic absorption of the drug. Its half life is 22 hours, making once a day dosing adequate.

Ezetimibe also blocks all other sterol absorption, making it the only effective treatment for sitosterolemia. Ezetimibe does not block the absorption of lipid-soluble vitamins or other medications. Ezetimibe is proven safe in HIV patients and is probably safe in renal patients.

Side effects

When used with a statin, ezetimibe can raise liver enzymes (so you need to monitor it) or cause muscle problems. Ezetimibe has even been reported to cause myopathy and rhabdomyolosis even when administered alone.

Contra-indications

The contra-indications include active liver disease, women who are pregnant or may become pregnant, nursing mothers, and known hypersensitivity.

PCSK9 Inhibitors

The enzyme PCSK9 (proprotein convertase subtilisin/kexin type 9) plays an important role in regulating the LDL receptor (LDL-R). The LDL-R is expressed on the surface of hepatocytes and possesses a specific binding domain for apolipoprotein B (apoB), which is a component of circulation chylomicrons, VLDL, IDL, and LDL lipoproteins. After the apoB containing particle binds to the LDL-R, the complex undergoes endocytosis via a clathrin-coated pit. Once the LDL-R/ApoB complex is encased within the acidic confines of the endosome, the LDL-R conformation is altered and subsequently dissociates from the ApoB particle, the latter of which undergoes degradation to release its cholesterol contents. The fate of the LDL-R at that time is two-fold: it may either be recycled back to the cell surface to continue clearing ApoB-containing particles from circulation, or be targeted for degradation.

The enzyme PCSK9 controls whether LDL-R continues to recycle or is degraded within the cell. If PCSK9 is not attached to the LDL-R/apoB complex, the LDL-R is released intact and recycles to the cell surface, where it continues to remove ApoB. If and when the PCSK9 attaches to the LDL-R/apoB complex, the shape of the complex is altered and the entire complex is degraded. This degradation process catabolizes the LDL-R. Essentially PCSK9 reduces the number of functioning LDL-R, which in turn increases the level of circulating cholesterol. Remember: increased PCSK9 activity leads to fewer LDL-R so higher serum cholesterol levels. If PCSK9 activity is reduced or blocked, then the LDL-R/apoB/PCSK9 complex does not form, LDL-R are not degraded, the LDL-R recycle continuing to remove cholesterol from the circulation, and the serum cholesterol level is lower.

Illustration 15 LDL-R recycles (left-hand side) removing cholesterol from circulation unless PCSK9 attaches to the LDL-R/apoB complex which leads to the degradation of LDL-R (right-hand side)

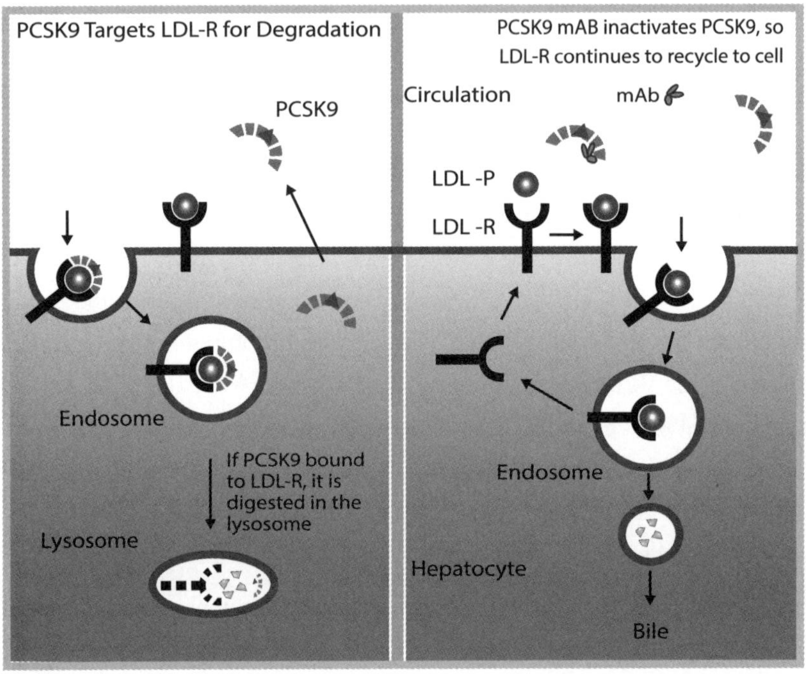

There are additional cellular mechanisms at play in the regulation of LDL-R expression. Sterol regulatory element-binding protein (SREBP), which is a transcription factor, increases HMG CoA-reductase and LDL-R gene expression in the response to low intracellular cholesterol levels. By inhibiting the activity of HMG CoA reductase, intracellular cholesterol levels are reduced in the setting of statin use. This reduction in cholesterol stimulates a counter-regulatory effect by SREBP-related transcription of LDL-R and PCSK9. While the upregulation in LDL-R helps to further augment LDL-C clearance from circulation and boost intracellular cholesterol stores, the concomitant increase in PCSK9 renders a certain percentage of

LDL-R ineffective in further binding to ApoB containing particles. This counter-regulatory increase in PCSK9 has been observed with statin use, as well as fibrate and ezetimibe use. Taken together, the consequent rise of PCSK9 levels following treatment with current lipid-lowering drugs allows for an additive, and synergistic, role seen with the use of PCSK9 inhibitors.

The monoclonal antibodies, alirocumab and evolocumab (both recently approved by the FDA) and bocozcizumab, attach to different epitopes of PCSK9, thereby inhibiting the binding to the LDL-receptor, which prevents the degradation of receptor in the hepatocyte and allows the LDL-R to recycle back to the cell surface. Therefore, anti-PCSK9 monoclonal antibodies (mAbs) improve LDL receptor upregulation, resulting in lower LDL-C levels.

These new medications have significant potential to lower LDL-C in patients who are at very high risk (e.g., those with Familial Hypercholesterolemia or known CAD) but not able to reach goal.

At this time, the FDA indications for the PCSK9 inhibitors are

- Alirocumab is indicated "as an adjunct to diet and maximally tolerated statin therapy for the treatment of adults with heterozygous familial hypercholesterolemia or clinical atherosclerotic cardiovascular disease, who require additional lowering of LDL-cholesterol."
- Evolocumab is indicated as an adjunct to diet and maximally tolerated statin therapy for the treatment of adults with heterozygous Familial Hypercholesterolemia or clinical atherosclerotic disease, who require additional lowering of LDL-cholesterol, and other LDL-lowering therapies (e.g., statins, ezetimibe, apheresis) in patients with homozygous familial hypercholesterolemia (HoFH) who require additional lowering of LDL-C.

They offer enormous LDL-C reductions of 50% to 60% when used alone or in conjunction with background statin and non-statin therapies with benefits seen across subgroups in clinical trials. At this time, numerous phase 1–3 trials have shown their efficacy in lowering LDL, with suggestions of potential CV event reductions based upon a very limited amount of post hoc or prespecified analyses.

Despite their subcutaneous route of administration, PCSK9 inhibitors appear to be well-tolerated with an acceptable side effect profile. Most of the statistically significant side effects are linked to reactions to the injection agents and not the medication (e.g., sore throat, injection site reactions, nasopharyngitis, and itching). Special attention is being paid to the possibility of cognitive effects with their use, but there is no definitive evidence of this based on the current data.

The initial indication for anti-PCSK9 mAb is for patients on maximally tolerated statins with heterozygous familial hypercholesterolemia or atherosclerotic cardiovascular disease who require additional LDL-C reduction. Clinical judgment is warranted to determine which patients require additional LDL-C lowering. In light of the recent IMPROVE-IT trial supporting the "lower is better" hypothesis, clearly the patient population with LDL-C > 100 mg/dl with atherosclerotic cardiovascular disease is the subgroup of trial subjects that have been shown to have benefits from intensive statin therapy and therefore are patients who also are likely to have improved outcomes with anti-PCSK9 therapy even on maximally tolerated statins.

As the future outcome studies are published, these exciting new medications will give us new insights into our understanding of what it takes to further and significantly lower CAD events and mortality and our understanding of LDL-C pathogenesis of atherosclerosis.

Medications that lower triglyceride

Niacin

Niacin, a member of the vitamin B3 family, has several powerful lipid-altering effects when used in large doses. Historically, the chief indications for niacin are hyper-triglyceridemia or combination therapy for the treatment of the atherogenic dyslipidemia seen with insulin resistance.

However, the AIM-HIGH study concluded that when patients were given high-intensity statin (LDL < 70), the addition of niacin did not produce additional clinical benefit despite improvements in HDL-C and triglyceride levels.

Mechanism of action

Niacin has several favorable lipid-altering actions. Niacin reduces hepatic formation of VLDL-P by reducing the mobilization of free fatty acids from peripheral adipose tissue. Niacin binds to the niacin receptor on the adipocyte, which blocks the release of free fatty acids (FFA). Since FFA is the substrate for triglyceride synthesis in the liver, less triglyceride production leads to decreased secretion of VLDL. Second, niacin probably up-regulates ABCA-1, which transfers free cholesterol from macrophages to nascent apo A-1 to start the process of reverse cholesterol transfer. Niacin also may raise HDL-C by decreasing the catabolism of HDL-P. By decreasing VLDL secretion, less triglyceride is available for transfer from HDL-P to VLDL via CETP. This keeps the HDL-P relatively cholesterol enriched and triglyceride poor. These large cholesterol-enriched particles are more slowly catabolized than small triglyceride-rich HDL.

Therapeutic uses of niacin

Niacin lowers elevated triglycerides by 20% to 50%, lowers LDL-C by 5% to 20%, and increases HDL-C by 15% to 35%. Niacin will also lower Lp(a) by 25%, decrease fibrinogen levels by 15% to 50%, and decrease Lp-PLA-2—also all good things for preventing and reducing CVD, particularly in dyslipidemic patients.

The effects of niacin on the major lipids are dose dependent, as shown in the following table.

Table 28 The effect of niacin on lipids is dose dependent
Numbers in percent

Daily dose	LDL-C	TG	HDL-C
Niacin 1000	No effect	↓ 25 to 30	↑ 25 to 30
Niacin 2000	↓ 10 to 15	↓ 35 to 50	↑ 25 to 30

Importantly, by reducing free fatty acid mobilization and lowering triglycerides, niacin also has favorable secondary effects on the TG/HDL axis disorders seen with insulin resistance. As the TG falls, CETP activity is slowed. This makes (1) the LDL-P larger so they are more easily recognized by LDL-R and removed from circulation, (2) the HDL-P larger so the apo A-1 is not excreted in the urine and remain in circulation where they can restart reverse cholesterol transport, and (3) both apo B and non-HDL decrease.

The various niacins

Sorry, but the multiple types of "niacin" are a tad complex. Much of the confusion arises because niacin refers to a whole group of chemicals ranging from over-the-counter vitamins to high-potency prescription medications, some of which cause flushing and others liver damage. These niacin compounds are not interchangeable and do not have the same effect on lipids. Even more confusing, those niacins that do improve lipids have different metabolisms and different adverse effect profiles.

First, let's list and dispense with the products that have no effect on lipids: vitamin B3, niacinamide, and inositol nicotinate. These over-the-counter "niacins" do not produce a flush and have no beneficial effect on lipids.

The lipid-altering niacins all cause flushing. The side effects and efficacy of these effective niacin compounds are related to their rate of intestinal absorption and which of two hepatic pathways metabolize which niacin. One hepatic pathway has a high capacity, but the niacin metabolites minimize flushing. The other hepatic pathway does not cause flushing but has a low capacity that can be overloaded, leading to liver toxicity.

Immediate-release niacin follows the high-capacity pathway and minimizes the risk of liver toxicity, but does cause substantial flushing. The controlled-release niacin compounds (synonyms include slow-, controlled-, sustained-, time-release-, long-acting-) were designed for slow absorption so as not to overload the low-capacity liver pathways and to minimize flushing. Unfortunately, many slow-release niacins formulations minimize flushing at the expense of reduced lipid efficacy and an increased incidence of hepatic toxicity. The newest extended-release niacin preparation seeks a middle path that minimizes both liver toxicity and flushing while maximizing the lipid effect.

In summary: immediate-release niacin saturates the liver pathway quickly so the remainder of the drug causes flushing. Slow-release niacin does not cause flushing because it is slowly being metabolized by, but not saturating, the liver pathway. Extended-release niacin was designed to balance these two pathways; it causes a little flushing with the benefit of a reduced risk of liver disease.

The take-home lesson is that these niacin medications may not be taken interchangeably. Use a prescription niacin, either immediate-release niacin or extended-release niacin (Niaspan). We also recommend that you strongly advise your patients to not switch their niacin medication to over-the-counter niacins and to let you know if they are taking a slow-release niacin. If a patient is taking an immediate-release niacin, give them a drug holiday of about 10 days before starting extended-release niacin.

Side Effects

All niacin compounds that lower lipids and lipoproteins cause flushing in nearly all patients. This flushing is prostaglandin-mediated, temporary, not life-threatening, and can be reduced by taking an anti-inflammatory 30 to 60 minutes before the taking the niacin. Tachyphylaxis will develop in about six weeks. This flushing may be as close to a menopausal hot flash as most men experience—tell them it's only a hot flash; they won't die.

Niacin may also raise slightly a fasting blood sugar, particularly in patients who have insulin resistance. Unfortunately, this is exactly where the drug is most effective and often most necessary.

Recommendations of the NLA

The National Lipid Association Safety Committee has the following recommendations for patients with impaired fasting glucose or diabetes:

Patients with normal fasting glucose

Niacin may be used, but minor increases of glucose may occur.

Patients with IFG or IGT without diabetes

Either defer niacin while controlling the IFG and/or IGT or start niacin with close glucose monitoring. This is the area where niacins are most beneficial by affecting the misaligned TG/HDL axis.

Patients with type 2 diabetes

Niacin is most helpful in the management of patients with diabetic dyslipidemia and should be used. Blood sugars should be monitored and anti-glycemic medications adjusted as necessary.

Other side effects

Niacin may also cause dyspepsia with worsening of peptic ulcer disease, hyperuricemia with development or worsening of gout, cystoid macular edema, atrial fibrillation, and acanthosis nigrans. And importantly, there is a small risk that niacin may increase the risk of myopathy if used with a statin.

Contra-indications and warnings

The contra-indications to Niaspan include active liver disease, active peptic ulcer disease, arterial bleeding (as if we see that in a lipid or preventive cardiology clinic!), and the usual known hypersensitivity.

The "warnings" section of the product package insert is informative, as always. The warnings include (1) "severe hepatic toxicity has occurred in patients substituting sustained-release niacin for immediate-release niacin at equivalent doses, (2) myopathy when co-administered with a statin in the elderly, or patients with renal failure, diabetes, or uncontrolled hypothyroidism, (3) liver enzyme elevations, (4) use with caution in patients with angina or during an acute phase of an MI, and (5) glucose monitoring."

Hints to prescribing niacins successfully

To minimize the flushing reactions associated with niacin, follow these helpful steps:

1. Always start niacin slowly and titrate upward at four week intervals. If patients stop the niacin for whatever reason, they need to start the titration again. Tachyphylaxis develops over about six weeks, but is lost quickly if the niacin is stopped for more than a day or two.
2. Take 325 mg of aspirin or 200 of an NSAID 30 minutes before taking the niacin.
3. Take the niacin with a low-fat food.
4. Do not eat spicy food or drink alcohol or hot beverages with the niacin.

Despite these instructions, an estimated 10% of your patients will find the flushing intolerable.

At baseline, then at 6 to 8 weeks, and then every 6 months check LFTs, fasting glucose, and uric acid.

Fibrates

Fibrates have been used to treat lipid disorders for nearly 50 years. In both primary and secondary trials, they reduce atherosclerosis and coronary events by lowering triglycerides and raising HDL-C.

Fibrates are primarily beneficial in patients with elevated triglycerides, or the borderline triglycerides and decreased HDL-C seen with metabolic syndrome and atherogenic dyslipidemia. They are even more effective in the group with low HDL-C and either pre-diabetes or actual type 2 diabetes.

Mechanism

Fibrates have many actions, all of which are beneficial. They lower triglycerides by stimulating PPARα, which increases fatty acid uptake and oxidation, reducing the hepatic substrate necessary to make triglycerides, and they stimulate LPL and inhibit apo C-III. The net effect is a decrease in all TG-rich lipoproteins.

Fibrates have many other salutatory effects. They increase and improve HDL. They stimulate apo A-1, which increases the production of HDL-P; they increase ABCA-1, which loads the apo A-1 with cholesterol from a macrophage; and they stimulate SR-B1, which pulls more cholesterol ester from the HDL-P into the liver as part of reverse cholesterol transport.

Fibrates are anti-inflammatory. They reduce NF-KB, IL-6, fibrinogen, endothelial adhesion molecules, and metalloproteinases. And fibrates raise adiponectin improving insulin sensitivity.

Effects of Fibrates

Fibrates are primarily used to lower triglycerides. They usually lower triglyceride levels by 30% to 50%. If the triglycerides are below 400, the LDL-C either stays the same or falls about 10%. However, if the triglycerides are over 400, the LDL-C often increases. Fibrates may also raise the HDL 5% to 20%. Fibrates are particularly effective in mixed dyslipidemia when used in conjunction with a statin.

The two major fibrates, gemfibrozil and fenofibrate (along with its active form, fenofibric acid) have different non-lipid effects and dosing in renal failure.

Side effects of the fibrates

The two different classes of fibrates have a strikingly different effect when given with statins. Here we mean gemfibrozil on one hand and, on the other, fenofibric acid, which is the active metabolite of fenofibrate.

If possible, gemfibrozil should not be used in combination with statins because it competes for the glucuronidation process with statins. The fibric acid fibrates do not compete for glucuronidation and have a much safer use profile with statins.

Fibrates have been associated with slightly increased risks for cholelithiasis, venous thrombosis, and perhaps an increase in non-cardiovascular mortality when given to patients who do not have starting elevations of triglycerides or lowered levels of HDL-C.

Fibrates may increase the serum creatinine modestly, but this effect is not associated with any increased risk of renal failure. And, although the clinical effect is not clear, fibrates may increase the homocysteine.

Contra-indications to fibrates

Fibrates are contra-indicated in nursing mothers and in patients who have gallbladder disease or active liver disease. The fenofibrate and fenofibric acid have dose limitations in renal disease, but gemfibrozil may be used in these same patients without dose restriction.

Myopathies, including rhabdomyolysis, have been reported in patients taking fibrates and statins. Fibrates also increase serum creatinine levels, but this does appear to have clinical significance.

Fibrates and renal failure

The National Kidney Foundation also recommends the following maximum doses by GFR for other lipid medications.

Table 29 Fibrate dose by GFR
Doses are in mg

	90 +	60 to 90	30 to 59	< 30
Fenofibrate	201	134	67	Avoid
Gemfibrozil	600 bid	600 bid	600 bid	600 bid
Niacin	1000	1000	1000	

Omega-3 fatty acids EPA and DHA

Omega-3 fatty acids are cardio-protective in a multitude of ways. The data clearly shows that omega-3 fatty acids reduce sudden death and lower triglycerides. They also improve endothelial function, are anti-inflammatory, and anti-thrombotic.

Mechanism

The multiple mechanisms of action for the omega-3 fatty acids EPA and DHA are not clearly understood. Omega-3 fatty acids lower triglycerides by reducing the synthesis of triglycerides in the liver and by increasing LPL activity, which increases hydrolysis.

Effects

Omega-3 fatty acids refer to the two cardio-protective fatty acids, EPA and DHA. EPA and DHA reduce triglycerides in a dose-dependent manner; reduce the risk of sudden death; improve endothelial function by increasing nitric oxide; and are anti-inflammatory by reducing cytokines, interleukins, and TNF.

The American Heart Association has clear recommendations for the use of omega-3 fatty acids EPA and DHA.

Patients without CVD (That means everyone who does not already have heart disease.)

> Eat a deep-water ocean fish at least twice a week and include foods rich in α-linolenic acid (e.g., flaxseed, canola or soybean oil, and walnuts). Alternatively, everyone should take a daily supplement that contains at least 500 mg of EPA and DHA combined.

Patients with CVD

> Get one gram of EPA/DHA daily from either fatty fish or a capsule containing one gram of EPA/DHA.

Please note that 1,000 mg of "fish oil" does not mean that the pill contains 1,000 mg of the cardioprotective EPA and DHA. Most OTC fish oils contain only a small quantity of the active ingredients EPA and DHA. Your patients must look at the active ingredients list on the label and be certain they are getting adequate doses of EPA plus DHA. Tell your patients to buy only fish oils that contain adequate amounts of DHA plus EPA, or give them a prescription omega-3.

Omega-3 fatty acids will lower triglycerides and non-HDL (the sum of all atherogenic lipoproteins), may minimally increase HDL, and may raise LDL-C. Importantly, using a high-intensity omega-3 to lower triglycerides does not change PCSK9 activity (unlike the fibrates).

Omega-3 fatty acids lower triglyceride in a dose-dependent manner. These doses require prescription-strength omega-3s.

Side effects

The side effects of omega-3 fatty acids are minimal, limited to burping and dyspepsia. There is some risk of excess bleeding. Omega-3 fatty acids do not affect the AUC and C_{max} of statin, do not increase fasting glucose, and do not interfere with any other lipid-lowering medications.

Names

Omega-3 fatty acids are often confused with "fish oil," which just happens to be where they are most commonly found. However, "fish oil" on the label does not necessarily mean that much of the healthy EPA and DHA are inside the pills. Many "fish oils" contain as little as 200 mg of EPA/DHA in each "1,000 mg capsule."

There are three FDA-approved prescription omega-3 fatty acids: Lovaza and Epanova each contain 750–850 mg of purified EPA/DHA per capsule. Vascepa contains pure EPA. Lovaza and Vascepa are in the ethyl ester form, which is digested into a free fatty acid prior to absorption, which requires significant pancreatic lipase activity. Epanova is already in the free fatty acid form and therefore has improved biovailability compared to the ethyl ester formulations, thereby allowing for a lower dose (2 grams per day rather than 4 grams for Lovaza or Vascepa).

Medications to raise HDL-C

HDL is important in reverse cholesterol transport, the process of carrying cholesterol away from the intima and back to the liver. Numerous studies point to the benefit of raising the level of HDL-C, especially in those patients with sub-optimal levels. For each 1 mg increase in HDL-C, the risk of CVD falls by 2% or 3%.

The power of exercise to increase the HDL is well-known. A meta-analysis of 95 exercise studies found that exercise led to a 6% decline in total cholesterol, 10% decline in LDL-C, and a 5% increase in HDL-C. (Tran *JAMA* 1985; 254: 919–924) Exercise appears to be most beneficial if it is aerobic, totals more than 30 minutes a day (in a minimum of 10-minute aliquots), and is equivalent to or greater than brisk walking.

Unfortunately, trials with medications to raise HDL have not been successful. We now know that even adding niacin to a high-intensity statin in an effort to raise the HDL does not lead to better outcomes. And all of the published CTEP inhibitor trials have failed.

To raise the HDL, it is best to stick with statins and lifestyle: daily activity equaling 30 minutes of brisk walking, a diet that avoids transfats and emphasizes fruits and veggies, and no smoking.

Combining Lipid Medications

Many patients require more than one medication to control their lipid disorder. This includes patients with dyslipidemia, metabolic syndrome, and the familial lipid disorders.

The primary starting medication for almost all patients with a lipid disorder is a statin, because it has been shown conclusively to reduce CVD events and mortality. We have organized this section assuming that you are adding something to a statin. It is also quite permissible to add two non-statin lipid-lowering medications together and these combinations are shown in the therapeutic and protocol chapter.

Adding ezetimibe to a statin

Taken together, the evidence clearly shows 1) that any lowering of LDL is more beneficial than not and 2) that even lower is even better. The chart below shows a plot line between the results of several statin studies with the results observed for both the study placebo and study drug outcomes. Note how well the IMPROVE-IT study showed that the addition of ezetimibe to a statin fit on the curve. Keep in mind that IMROVE-IT compared two groups: one on a statin with an average LDL of 69 and the other on statin plus ezetimibe with an average LDL of 53.

Chart 5 Relative risk of CAD plotted against LDL values on placebo and treatment arms of various studies show that lower is better

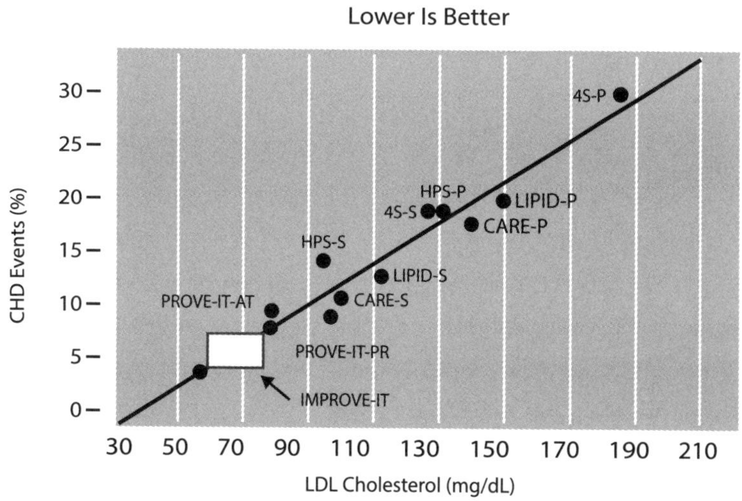

Adding ezetimibe to a statin is a potent method to further and consistently lower the LDL with minimal increased side effects.

Adding ezetimibe to a statin is often the best way to achieve that goal.

The recent IMPROVE-IT trial shows that the addition of ezetimibe decreases the LDL-C by an additional 20% and the relative risk of CAD by 6%. This effect is exactly the same as going from the lowest to highest dose of a statin (e.g., ezetimibe 10 added to simva 10 gets the same LDL-C lowering as going from simva 10 to to 80) and without the added potential risks associated with a highest-dose statin. Adding ezetimibe to a statin carries a slightly increased risk of elevated LFTs which should be check periodically. Combining ezetimibe and a statin does not appear to increase the risk of myopathy but does have the potential to increase myalgias.

Adding a bile acid sequestrant to a statin

Adding bile acid sequestrants to a statin further lowers the LDL-C. Both medications work on different mechanisms on the LDL-C side of the equation. Additionally, one of the bile acid sequestrants, colesevelam, has an FDA indication to "improve glycemic control in adults with type 2 diabetes."

Colesevelam is thus helpful in our diabetic patients, all of whom will already be on statins by guideline.

Bile acid sequestrants require two reminders: first, adding a bile acid sequestrant to a statin will increase the triglycerides; and, in fact, adding BAS is contra-indicated if the triglycerides are above 400. Second, you need to separate the dose of the BAS and the many medications.

Adding niacin to a statin

Niacin was once considered a potent addition to statins, especially in patients with the "residual cardiovascular risk" seen with metabolic syndrome (e.g., the persistent elevation of LDL-P, elevated triglycerides, and lower HDL despite statin therapy to a good LDL level). However, two recent large trials, AIM-HIGH and HPS2-THRIVE, failed to show outcomes benefit from the addition of niacin to a statin. Even more troubling, adding niacin to statin seemed to increase adverse events.

For these reasons, the addition of niacin to a statin has fallen out of favor and is no longer recommended. Niacin is still a fine drug by itself and has benefit, just no additional benefit when added to a statin.

Adding a fibrate to a statin

As with adding niacin to a statin, the addition of a fibrate to a statin covers two sides of the lipid disorders: statins lower LDL-C and fibrates lower triglycerides. It is important to note that fibrates lower LDL-P and apo B only modestly or not at all in combination with a statin in patients with hypertriglyceridemia.

If the starting triglycerides are above about 400, the addition of a fibrate may actually increase the LDL-C. This happens because the fibrate increases the LPL activity which increases the conversion of VLDL-C to LDL-C. LDL-P and Apo B are not increased and may slightly decrease.

We must note that adding a fibrate to a statin increases the risk of rhabdomyolysis. But the risk with the addition of gemfibrozil is much greater than with the addition of a fenofibrate or fenofibric acid, and the worst offending statin, cerivastatin, has been withdrawn from the market. Fibrates also raise

PCSK9 levels which may aggravate the LDL-C increase in combination with statins, especially high-dose statins which significantly increase PCSK9 upregulation.

Fibrates and statins both have pleotropic effects including improved endothelial function, reduced inflammation, and the stabilization of plaques. In addition, fibrates have a positive effect on microvascular complications of type 2 diabetes.

Choosing whether to add niacin or fibrates to a statin

Niacins and fibrates have a similar use and effect on the lipoprotein panel. However, there are a couple of unique situations where one drug may be better than the other. For example, niacin increases uric acid, while fenofibrate and fenofibric acid lower uric acid. And niacin will increase the blood sugar while fenofibrates will improve blood sugars and prevent complications of microvascular disease in type 2 diabetes.

Adding high-dose omega-3 to a statin

High-dose omega-3s (e.g., 3 or 4 grams per day) will lower triglycerides. This, like niacin and fibrates, becomes an additional treatment for patients with both elevated cholesterol and triglycerides. As with niacin and the fibrates, the triglycerides and non-HDL will fall. If the TGs are elevated, the addition of omega-3s will effectively lower VLDL-C and non-HDL-C but may raise the LDL-C but not the LDL-P or apo B. Based on limited data to date, omega-3s, unlike fibrates, do not raise PSCK9 levels (which can offset the effects of a statin) and therefore appear to have a better non-HDL-C-lowering effect in combination with high-dose statins. Since Omega-3s have potential cardiovascular benefits, this therapy should be a consideration in patients on a statin with triglyceride greater than 200 mg and non-HDL-C not at goal.

Chapter 10

The Cardiometabolic Patient

We could not write this book without addressing the current pandemic of the metabolic syndrome, the diseaseproducing cluster of abdominal obesity, dyslipidemia, insulin resistance, and hypertension. Almost fifty million Americans have metabolic syndrome. Interestingly, 10% to 20% of patients with cardiometabolic risk are not obese but do have elevated triglycerides, depressed HDL-C, hypertension, and/or impaired fasting glucose. You can often identify metabolic syndrome by looking at the lipid panel; it shows atherogenic dyslipidemia: elevated triglycerides, a depressed HDL-C, and increased non-HDL (more than 30 mg above the LDL). If you do other lipid tests, you will see increased apo B, LDL-P, non-HDL-C, with depressed HDL-C levels, and increased numbers of small, dense LDL-P, often with near normal LDL-C levels.

Table 30 Biochemical problems associated with metabolic syndrome

Metabolic risk factors	Commonly measured components
Dyslipidemia	Elevated triglycerides Low HDL-C Elevated non-HDL-C, apo B, and LDL-P
Insulin resistance	Elevated fasting blood sugar Borderline A-1C
Prothrombotic state	High fibrinogen Plasminogen activator inhibitor PAI-1
A pro-inflammatory state	Elevated hsCRP

Some experts have questioned the use of the phrase "metabolic syndrome," preferring instead to focus on the individual components (dyslipidemia, hypertension, and type 2 diabetes). We support the use of the term "metabolic syndrome" to describe that particular patient who is so often seen in clinic, because this one clinical descriptive diagnosis should prompt the clinician to think of all the steps necessary for global risk management.

The definition of metabolic syndrome includes (1) visceral adiposity in most, but not all, patients and the associated dyslipidemia (2) low HDL-C, (3) elevated triglycerides with normal LDL-C, (4) hypertension, and (5) insulin resistance. The international criteria require obesity plus two other components; NCEP says that metabolic syndrome can be diagnosed whenever three of the five components are present.

Table 31 Criteria for metabolic syndrome

	International Diabetes Federation Central obesity + ≥ 2 of HDL, Trig, BP, or FBS		NCEP ATP III with 2004 Update ≥ 3 of below	
Visceral obesity in row 1 or 2 below plus 2 of row 3 through 6	Men	Women	Men	Women
Europeans, East Mediterranean, Middle Eastern, and Sub-Saharan Africans	≥ 94 cm ≥ 37 in	≥ 80 cm ≥ 31.5 in	≥ 40 in	≥ 35 in
South Asians, Chinese, Japanese, First Nations, Ethnic South and Central Americans	≥ 90 cm ≥ 35.5 in	≥ 80 cm ≥ 31.5 in		
HDL-C	< 1.03 mmol/L < 40 mg/dL	< 1.3 mmol/L < 40 mg/dL	< 40 mg/dL	< 50 mg/dL
Triglycerides	> 1.7 mmol /L ≥ 150 mg/dL		≥ 150 mg/dL	
BP > 130/85 or BP treatment	> 130/85		≥ 130/85	
FBS	> 5.6 mmol/L or type 2 DM > 100 mg/dL		≥ 100 mg/dL	

The metabolic syndrome more than doubles the risk of cardiovascular disease and increases by five-fold the risk of type 2 diabetes. The obesity-driven metabolic syndrome is currently the leading cause of premature cardiovascular disease in much of the developed world. The mortality effect of the metabolic syndrome is large enough to reverse the gains produced by the decline in smoking. How tragic.

We will briefly discuss the importance and mechanisms of abdominal visceral (abdominal) obesity, the lipid problems associated with the metabolic syndrome, and tell you why these patients often require multiple medications to treat their lipid and lipoprotein problems.

The problem with visceral adipose tissue

Key points

- Visceral adipose tissue leads to both insulin resistance and increased fatty acid production, which lead to atherogenic dyslipidemia.
- Visceral adipose tissue is also pro-thrombotic and pro-inflammatory, both of which lead to increased endothelial damage.
- Taken together, this atherogenic dyslipidemia, insulin resistance, increased inflammation, and pro-thrombotic state lead to an increased risk of an aggressive atherosclerosis.

Visceral adipose tissue is metabolically active, in contrast to subcutaneous adipose tissue, which is relatively quiescent. Visceral adipose tissue does a whole myriad of metabolic things—all of them bad and all of them acting synergistically to promote premature atherosclerosis and type 2 diabetes. The single term that best captures this nefarious activity is "insulin resistance."

Under normal conditions, insulin (1) promotes the cellular uptake of glucose, (2) suppresses hepatic gluconeogenesis, (3) shifts skeletal muscle toward storage of energy, (4) stimulates lipoprotein and hepatic lipases, (5) stimulates the hepatic breakdown of apo B, and (6) suppresses hormone-sensitive lipase to reduce the release of FFA from adipose tissues. When a patient is insulin resistant, all of these biochemical functions are compromised.

The primary lipid abnormalities associated with the insulin resistance of visceral adiposity are (1) an over-production of FFAs leading to over-production of VLDL-P and (2) increased CETP activity (see illustration 4 on page 24) that changes the ratio of cholesterol and triglyceride inside each circulating lipoprotein.

Visceral adipose tissue is resistant to the anti-lipolytic activity of insulin resulting in a high lipolytic activity. The result is an increased release of free fatty acids (FFA) into the portal circulation, which leads to an excess of free fatty acids in the liver. Free fatty acids in the liver are the primary driver of VLDL-P production or; when that capacity is overloaded, they are stored in the liver causing fatty liver.

This excess VLDL- P production quickly elevates the plasma triglyceride level. This in turn increases the activity of the CETP enzyme, which exchanges triglyceride in the VLDL-P for cholesterol in IDL-P, LDL-P, and HDL-P. Note that the serum total cholesterol level does not change; the cholesterol is simply transferred from one lipoprotein to another by CETP.

Unfortunately, this CETP-facilitated transfer has two atherosclerosis-promoting actions in the plasma.

First, this CETP-activated transfer process makes the LDL-P carry more triglyceride and less cholesterol ester. This induces further LDL-P lipolysis by hepatic lipase, making the LDL-P so small and misshapen that the LDL-R does not recognize and remove it. The patient now has numerous small, dense cholesterol-poor LDL-P that stay in the circulation for several days, attaching to the endothelium, where they are internalized and oxidized.

Second, the CETP-activated transfer process also decreases the cholesterol and increases the triglyceride in HDL-P. This triglyceride-rich HDL-P now undergoes further lipolysis by hepatic lipase, getting smaller in size, until the apo A-1 breaks free and is urinated away. And, that is why people with metabolic syndrome have low levels of HDL-P.

Identifying the lipid abnormalities of atherogenic dyslipidemia

You can suspect atherogenic dyslipidemia of insulin resistance when you see (1) a normal LDL-C but low HDL-C and even a minimally elevated triglyceride, (2) a TG/HDL > 3.5, (3) a normal LDL-C but an elevation of non-HDL-C, (4) an HDL below 40 in men and 50 in women, or (5) an elevated fasting blood sugar.

LDL-C is less predictive of atherosclerosis and adverse cardiovascular events than non-HDL-C, apo B or LDL-P. Even worse, in atherogenic dyslipidemia, the discordance between the LDL-C and the lipoprotein apo B particles is often substantial, with the particles at a much higher population percentile than the cholesterol.

Lipid and lipoprotein discordance in atherogenic dyslipidemia

Patients with the metabolic syndrome and atherogenic dyslipidemia often have a substantial disconnect between their LDL-C and both the apo B or LDL-P. These patients may have normal LDL-C levels but very high levels of the B lipoproteins—and it is the particles that enter the arterial intima that start the atherosclerosis process.

As the triglycerides rise above somewhere between 100 and 150, the CETP enzyme begins to exchange the triglyceride in VLDL-P for the cholesterol ester in the apo B particles. This exchange loads the LDL-P with triglyceride, which then undergoes further hydrolysis, which makes the LDL-P smaller. These small, dense LDL-P are not recognized and removed by the LDL-R so they accumulate in the circulation where they have more opportunities to attach to the endothelium and cause atherosclerosis.

Cromwell and Otvos have a very clear chart showing the divergence between LDL-C and LDL-P as the triglyceride rises. Please note that this divergence starts right around a triglyceride of 100. (Cromwell, *Cur Athero Reports* 2004; 6: 381–387). This highlights the importance of paying attention to even modest increases in triglycerides (as we said above, "it's the company they keep, not the trigs themselves").

Chart 6 LDL-P and LDL-C by triglyceride level in the Framingham Offspring Study (adapted from Cromwell, *Cur Athero Reports* 2004; 6: 381–387)

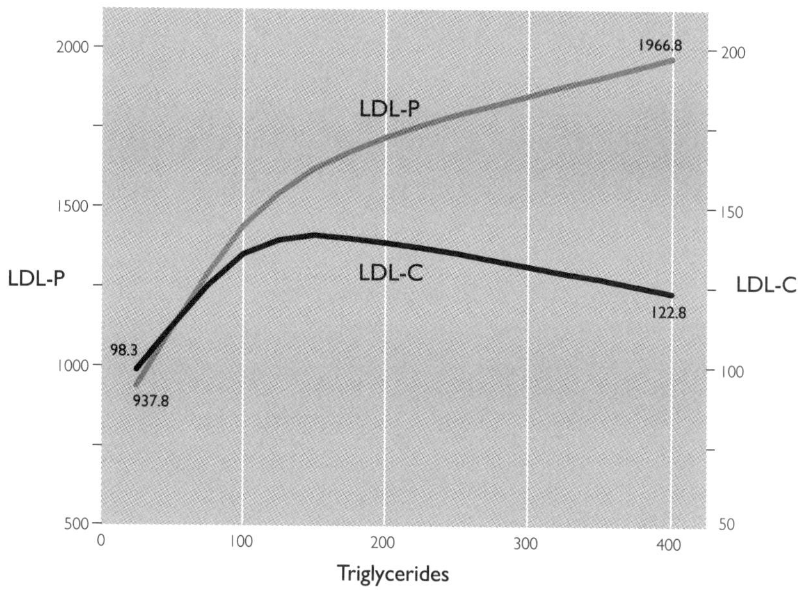

Cromwell et al. studied the lipoprotein particles of 3600 people in the Framingham Offspring Study and followed them for 14.8 years. They found that "LDL-P was a more sensitive indicator of CVD risks than either LDL-C or non-HDL-C." (Cromwell, J *Clin Lipid* 2007; 1: 583–592) This is shown in the following chart, which is taken from that same reference. Patients were divided into groups above or below the medians: the dividing median for LDL-C was 131 and the dividing median for LDL-P was 1414. Clearly, patients with less than the median LDL-P had better survival regardless of their LDL-C than did patients with a high LDL-P regardless of their LDL-C.

Chart 7 16-year survival by LDL-P and LDL-C in Framingham Offspring Study (adapted from Cromwell J *Clin Lipid,* 2007; 1: 583–592)

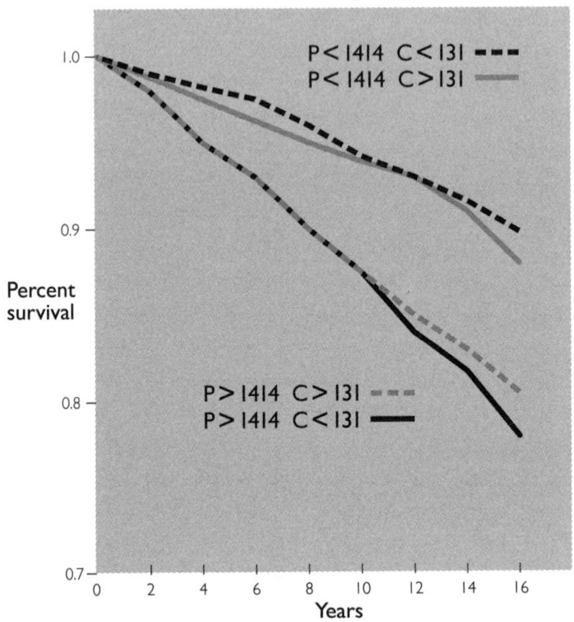

The visceral adipose tissue seen with cardiometabolic disease also secretes several chemicals that promote inflammation, coagulation, and atherosclerosis. These chemicals include the marker of systemic inflammation hsCRP, the pro-inflammatory IL-6, the pro-inflammatory tumor-necrosing factor-α TNF-α, the fibrinolysis inhibitor PAI-1, and resistin, which inhibits insulin activity.

Combine all of these viscerally-produced substances with the atherogenic dyslipidemia and an elevated fasting blood sugar and you get a real witch's brew. The inflammatory chemicals start to tear apart the endothelium and activate adhesion molecules, the numerous small IDL-P and LDL-P are pulled into the vascular intima, and other chemicals activate the oxidation process and macrophage endocytosis of the oxidized cholesterol. Even worse, the plaque is less stable because of increased metalloproteinase activity and any break in the plaque surface is more likely to encourage a propagating clot because fibrinolysis is inhibited. All too often, we call this disaster "sudden death."

If the patient has insulin resistance or cardiometabolic disease, he or she will often have:

1. A near normal LDL-C
2. Large size VLDL-P, which are filled with triglyceride. This explains the elevated levels of triglycerides, which drive the CETP transfer.
3. An increased circulating apo B count because all of the atherogenic lipoproteins are carrying abnormal ratios of triglyceride and cholesterol.
4. Large numbers of small, dense LDL-P. These are cholesterol poor and have a distorted apo B shape, which hinders uptake by hepatic LDL-R. It takes a great many small LDL-P to carry even normal amounts of LDL-C. This explains the normal serum LDL-C.
5. A depressed level of HDL-C. The action of CETP depletes HDL-P of cholesterol ester and fills the HDL-P with triglyceride. This, in turn, promotes the hepatic lipase activity, which leads to further hydrolysis, and this further reduces the HDL size, until the apo A-1 breaks free and is so small it can be excreted in the urine.
6. Increased inflammatory markers such as hsCRP.

Treating atherogenic dyslipidemia

Even early in the course of diagnosed disease, patients with the dyslipidemia of the metabolic syndrome often require lifestyle changes or multiple medications. Lifestyle changes are possible and will prevent the aggressive progression of disease. If patients fail to make lifestyle changes, then within a few years, many of them will be on two or three medications to treat their complex dyslipidemia, one or two drugs to treat their hypertension, and one or two drugs to treat their hyperglycemia and insulin resistance. Preventing this disease with lifestyle changes in the first place would be a whole lot cheaper and easier.

Early and aggressive treatment of abnormal lipids will lower CVD better than treating these patients after the diagnosis of CVD is made. Further, aggressively treating lipids has more clinical benefit than aggressively treating the hyperglycemia or borderline blood pressure. Per ACCORD, ADVANCE, and the VA Diabetes Trial, intensive glucose control does not reduce cardiovascular outcomes. Nonetheless, the best outcomes are seen in patients who do it all: make healthful lifestyle changes (daily exercise, weight loss, and healthy diet); and whose physicians treat their blood pressure, lipids, and blood sugars to the nationally recommended targets.

Expert opinion is divided on the target goals for treatment of patients with the metabolic syndrome and when to move a patient to the next treatment target. We expect further clarification from some of the soon-to-be-released national guidelines and we anticipate that these guidelines will move toward unified cutpoints and targets.

The American Diabetes Association and the American College of Cardiology recently issued a joint statement on the importance of lipoprotein management in patients with cardiometabolic risk. (Brunzell JD et al. *JACC* 2008; 51: 1521–1524 and *Diabetes Care* 2008; 31: 811–822)

- This consensus paper notes that LDL-C and non-HDL are the targets of current guidelines for those patients with cardiometabolic risk but without CVD or diabetes. Despite treatment with statins, these patients continue to have a significant residual risk of CVD due to elevated levels of apo B lipoproteins.
- The consensus statement calls for the measurement of apo B after LDL-C is lowered to target.
- The authors recommend that the highest-risk cardiometabolic risk patients (those who also have known CVD and those who do not yet have CVD but do have diabetes and one or more CMR factor beyond their dyslipidemia) be treated to an LDL-C < 70, a non-HDL-C < 100, and an apo B < 80. (These goals are nearly identical to those of the 2009 Canadian Consensus Statement for both moderate and high-risk patients.)

A 2005 study of 22,000 high-risk patients in various trials showed how far we are from hitting our apo B targets.

Table 32 Percentage of high-risk patients meeting goals study
(Stein EA *Am J Cardiol* 2005;96:36K-43K)

Subjects with triglycerides	LDL-C < 100 %	Non-HDL-C < 130 %	Apo B < 90 %
< 200	58	66	30
> 200	60	51	17

We must start with a strong emphasis on lifestyle changes because patients can eat and sit enough to overpower our medications. We must identify the correct target LDL-C and check that number as a population percentile, because that sets the goal for all other targets. Our therapeutic targets include getting the LDL-C, the non-HDL-C, apo B, or LDL-P to target. When choosing medications, and because of the primary target, you have several options: a statin powerful enough to achieve LDL-C goal, or a statin plus ezetimibe, or statin plus a fibrate, or statin plus niacin, or statin plus bile acid sequestrants.

Or, as is often necessary in patients with cardiometabolic disease, a combination of three or more drugs is necessary to gain control of the atherogenic dyslipidemia.

Chapter 11
CHECKLISTS FOR TREATING LIPID PATIENTS

WHEN PRESENTED WITH NEW patients or patients whose clinical status has changed, the first order of business is to determine whether they need lipid treatment; if so, ask both how aggressively they should be treated and what type of lipid problem they have and why.

Good lipid management requires a sequential process to efficiently and maximally reduce the burden of CVD without increasing risk to the patient of unnecessary treatment or testing. This chapter summarizes the steps that we follow in our active lipid clinics. These represent our best understanding of how to apply the current (multiple and conficiting) guidelines and science.

Cardiovascular disease could be better treated with better results if people follow this simple checklist. It is hard to believe, but we routinely see both patients with a stent or CABG or an LDL > 200 who are not on statins because the preventive cardiology checklist was not followed.

Step 1: Whom to treat?

- Patients who need immediate high-intensity treatment to LDL < 70 and non-HDL < 100. Treat, do not do any further stratification. Treatment will commonly take two lipid-lowering medications and/or newer therapies:

- Known atherosclerotic disease: CAD, PAD, CVA, CAC > 300, stents (frequently underplayed by the patient who says, "I don't have heart disease, just a stent."
- Patients over age 20 with Familial Hypercholesterolemia: LDL > 190 with family history of premature CAD or xanthomas (see Chapter 6).
    - If under age 45, reduce LDL by > 50%.
    - If > age 45, reduce LDL < 100.
    - If any other risk factors or existing disease, reduce LDL < 70.
- Patients with a Pooled Cohort Risk Calculator (or other calculator of your choice) with a ten-year risk > 15%.

► Patients who need or may need moderate-intensity statin treatment:
- Diabetics ages 40 to 75 with LDL 70 to 189.
- Patients with a Pooled Cohort Risk Calculator (or other calculator of your choice) with a ten-year risk > 7.5%.
- Patients (males > age 45, females > age 50) with multiple risk factors: any combination of diabetes, smoking, family history of first-degree relative with CAD < age 60, HDL < 40, Lp(a) > 100, CAC > 75th percentile, HIV, chronic inflammation, CKD stage 2 or 3.
- Patients with three or more of the criteria of metabolic syndrome, people of South Asian origin with a family history of premature CAD.

► Patients > age 45 (will have a low ten-year risk) who need further stratification, usually a coronary calcium scan. Treat with moderate intensity statin if CAC > 75th percentile using the MESA CAC calculator or treat with high-intensity statin if CAC > 300. Goal is < 100 unless they have more than one risk factor or if pre-existing disease, treat < 70.
- Patients with a strong family history of premature CAD < age 65, Lp(a) > 100, HDL < 40 but who are otherwise low-risk or < 7.5 ten-year risk on a calculator.

  - Patients with history of preeclampsia or erectile dysfunction.
  - Patients (males > age 45, females > age 50) with any risk factors:, smoking, family history of first-degree relative with CAD < age 60, HDL < 40, Lp(a) > 100, CAC > 75th percentile, HIV, chronic inflammation, CKD stage 2 or 3.
- Patients who are worried well
  - Lifestyle
  - LDL-lowering diet (see lifestyle Chapter 12) and consider stanols and sterols and/or red yeast rice.

Step 2: Treatment

- Lifestyle.
  - All patients, even those who do not require lipid management, should be counseled to follow a heart-healthy lifestyle with daily exercise, a heart-healthy diet, and no tobacco.
- High-intensity to LDL > 70 and non-HDL < 100:
  - Atorva 40 or 80 or rosuva 20 or 40.
  - If tolerating and not at goal, add ezetimibe.
  - If can only tolerate lower dose of a statin, then add ezetimibe and bile acid sequestrant or PCSK9 inhibitor if meet FDA criteria.
  - If intolerant of statins, refer to lipidologist for apheresis or novel therapies.
- Moderate-intensity statin:
  - Atorva 10 to 20
  - Fluva 40 bid or fluva XL 80
  - Lova 40
  - Pitava 2 to 4
  - Prava 40
  - Rosuva 5 to 10
  - Simva 20 to 40

If your target is other than LDL, use the table below to align the LDL target with non-HDL, LDL-P, or apoB. Note that it is often very difficult to get the LDL-P down to these percentiles levels, and there is no evidence that doing so improves outcomes.

Table 33 Treatment targets LDL-C goal percentile based on Framingham Offspring Study

Numbers rounded to nearest 5

NCEP Category	Target percentile	LDL-C	Non-HDL-C	LDL-P	Apo B
Very high risk	2	70	80	720	80*
High risk	20	100	120	1100	80
Moderately high risk	50	130	150	1440	95
Low risk	80	160	190	1820	120

* There is no real data to support getting an apo B below 80. At this time, an apo B target of 80 is sufficient even for the highest risk patients.

- Treat fasting triglycerides that exceed 750. The NLA says to treat if > 500, and the endocrine society says to treat with a fibrate if > 1,000.
  - Lifestyle is often more important than medications
  - If > 1500 a very low-fat diet is required
  - Otherwise diet recommendation is to limit fats, but almost more important is to limit sugars (esp. soda), refined flour, transfats, and processed foods
  - Lose weight, sometimes only 15 pounds is sufficient
  - If diabetic, get diabetes under better control
  - Limit alcohol
  - Omega 3 fatty acids, usually > 3 grams per day
  - Fenofibrates

Chart 8 The 2004 NCEP Risk Classification

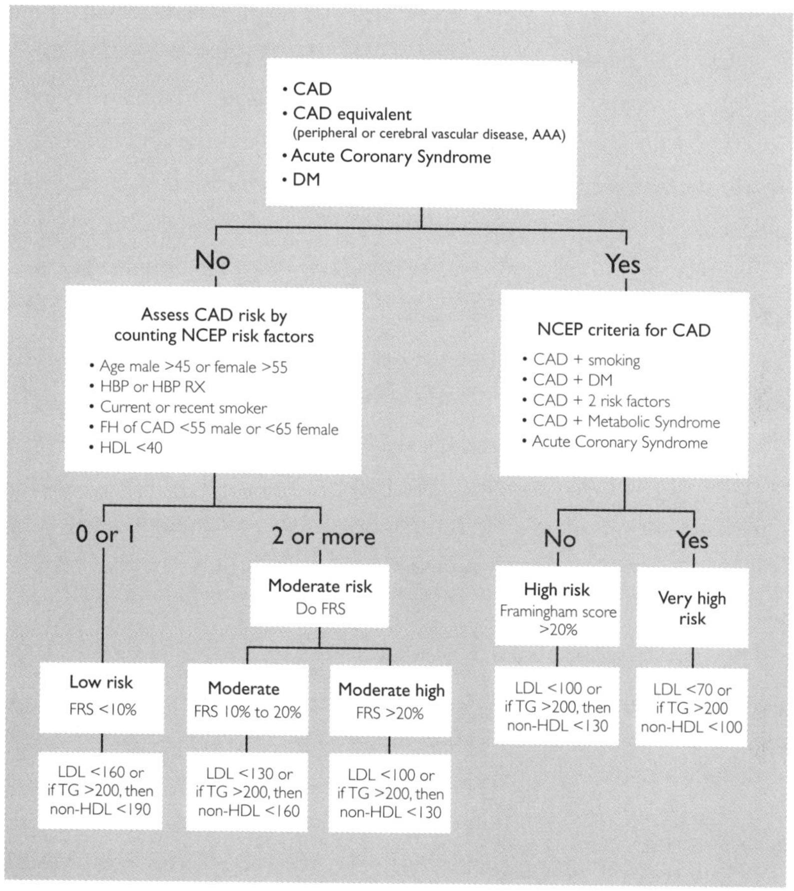

Checklist history and physical for a new lipid patient

The initial exam of a new or referral lipid patient has six goals: (1) to establish the presence of or risk for cardiovascular, (2) identify cardiovascular risk factors, (3) uncover any secondary causes of hyperlipidemia, (4) identify any genetic or lifestyle factors; (5) to calculate the ten-year risk and lipid goals; and (6) to start medication and lifestyle counseling.

In addition to the standard new patient history, a patient with primary lipid concerns should be asked about any first-degree relatives with premature cardiovascular disease. Familial combined hyperlipidemia (Fredrickson type IIb) is relatively common (1/200), presents in adulthood with modest elevations of total and LDL cholesterol and triglyceride, and substantially increases the risk of premature CVD in your patient. Family members should also be screened for lipid abnormalities.

The examination of a new lipid patient starts with measurement of height, weight, waist circumference, and calculation of BMI, pulse, BP, and respiratory rate. Because good lipid practitioners do not want to miss an important clue to the cause of the lipid disorder, they need to check each new patient for evidence of hypothyroidism, renal or hepatic disease, a corneal arcus or periorbital xanthomas, tendon xanthomas of the digital extensor tendons or Achilles, and any evidence of eruptive or palmar xanthomas.

Each patient deserves a good examination looking for physical evidence of cardiovascular disease.

Additional examinations may be necessary to determine the presence or absence of existing cardiovascular disease. These include a stress treadmill, carotid intimal medial thickness, ankle-brachial index, or coronary calcium measurement.

Checklist 1: Checklist for patients with elevated LDL-C, LDL-P, or non-HDL

1. Think about medical conditions
    a. Familial hypercholesterolemia
    b. Familial combined hypercholesterolemia
    c. Diabetes or pre-diabetes
    d. Hypothyroidism
    e. Renal disease
    f. Obstructive liver disease
    g. Anorexia nervosa

   h. HIV
   i. Cushings
   j. PCOS
   k. Pregnancy
2. Think about medications
   a. Anabolic steroids
   b. Cyclosporines
   c. Progestins
   d. Thiazides
   e. Fibrates if the initial trigs were elevated
   f. Niacin if the initial trigs were elevated
   g. Omega-3s if the initial trigs were elevated

Checklist 2: Checklist for patient with elevated trigs

1. Think about medical conditions
   a. Hyperchylomicronemia (trigs > 1000)
   b. Familial combined hypercholesterolemia
   c. Dysbetalipoproteinemia
   d. Familial hypertriglyceridemia
   e. Familial lipoprotein lipase deficiency (trigs > 1000)
   f. Insulin resistance
   g. Diabetes
   h. Lipodystrophy
   i. Gaucher's
   j. Hepatitis
   k. Chronic renal disease
   l. HIV
   m. Pregnancy
   n. A diet high in refined carbohydrates

2. Think about medications
    a. Bile acid sequestrants
    b. Estrogens
    c. Oral contraceptives
    d. SERMs
    e. Thiazides in high doses
    f. Cyclosporine
    g. Atypical anti-psychotics
    h. Steroids
    i. Protease inhibitors
    j. Long-term interferon

Checklist 3: Checklist for patients with low HDL

1. Think about medical conditions
    a. Insulin resistance
    b. Metabolic syndrome
    c. Smoking
    d. A high-carbohydrate diet
    e. A very low fat diet
2. Think about medications and substances
    a. Anabolic steroids
    b. Trans-fats
    c. Progestins
    d. Adding a glitazone to a fibrate (rare)
    e. Isoretinoids
    f. Beta blockers

The following strategy outlines medical blood tests that should be completed when a new lipid medication is started.

Strategy 1 Suggested laboratory tests at each step of lipid management

Before starting lipid Rx		
Lipids		Assess need for Rx and proper Rx
LFTs		Check for unexplained LFT elevation before starting Rx
FBS or A1C		Exclude diabetes
TSH		Exclude hypothyroidism
UA + Creatinine		Exclude acute and chronic renal disease
If starting or adding Rx		
	8 weeks after new Rx or dose change	**Maintenance**
Statin	Lipids AST ALT	Q 6 months Lipids Q 12 months lipids
Niacin	Lipids FBS ALT AST	Q 3 months for 1 year Lipids, AST, ALT, glucose Q 6 months Lipids, AST, ALT, glucose
Fibrate	Lipids FBS AST, ALT CBC	Q 6 months Lipids, AST, ALT, FBS, CBC
Ezetimibe	Lipids	LFTs at 8 weeks Q 6 months
BAS	Lipids	Q 3 months Lipids, FBS, Q 12 months Lipids, AST, ALT, FBS
Omega-3	Lipids FBS	Q 6 months Lipids

The attached strategies will walk you through a stepped approach to treatment and give you alternatives when the first treatments do not work or cannot be tolerated.

Strategy 2 Familial combined hyperlipidemia or Metabolic Syndrome

1. Check , FBS, A1C, or 2 hour blood sugar
   a. Emphasize importance of healthful lifestyle
      i. Mono-saturated and omega-3 fats >> saturated fats
      ii. Limit refined carbohydrates and alcohol
      iii. Emphasize colorful fruits and veggies, whole grains, and nuts
   b. Promote a minimum of 30 minutes of brisk walking every day
   c. Promote weight loss of 7% to 10% of body weight (the achieved weight loss of Diabetes Prevention Program)
   d. Monitor BP
   e. Consider sleep apnea
2. Start a mid-level dose of a high-potency statin
   Atorva 20
   Simva 20
   Rosuva 10 to 20
3. Recheck LDL-C, triglycerides, non-HDL-C, and apo B or LDL-P
   If any not at goal, then add either
   a. Fenofibrate 150 or fenofibric acid 120
      i. Use gemfibrozil only if renal failure present or formulary restrictions
   b. Omega-3
      i. The authors have the best results with the liquid omega-3, which contain > 1,750 mg of the active EPA + DHA
4. Recheck LDL-C, triglycerides, non-HDL-C, and apo B or LDL-P
   If still not at goals
   a. Start to combine the above medications
   b. Statin + fibrate + omega-3 (aim for maximal dose tolerated)
5. Recheck LDL-C, triglycerides, non-HDL-C, and apo B or LDL-P
   If still not at goals
   a. Start to combine the above medications
   b. Statin + fibrate + niacin (aim for maximal dose tolerated) + omega-3
   c. Recheck liver functions and blood sugar if started niacin

Strategy 3 Triglycerides > 500

For all patients with Triglycerides > 500

Look for underlying causes from checklist on page 134

Emphasize importance of healthful lifestyle

Low-fat diet is essential (see diet section for more notes)

Limit carbohydrates

Avoid alcohol

Promote daily exercise, at least 30 minutes of brisk walking

Check liver enzymes, uric acid and fasting blood sugar or A1C

Check FBS, A1C or 2-hour blood sugar

By definition, the target TG is < 150, so full doses of medications are often required

1. Start with fenofibrate, fenofibric acid, or omega-3 4 grams (Epanova 2 grams as an option). If you are likely to add a statin later, avoid gemfibrozil unless renal failure or formulary requirements
2. If trigs > 1,500, start fenofibric acid 145 and prescription omega-3 at a dose of 4 grams simultaneously
3. Add moderate dose of a high-strength statin (atorva, rosuva, and simva have specific indication for elevated trigs). Use caution if you use both gemfibrozil and a statin
4. Add one of the drugs you did not use at start to the above
5. Add the remaining drugs to the above combination

Strategy 4 Statin-intolerant patients

Step 1. Statins have proven efficacy to lower the CVD associated with elevated LDL-C, so staying with a statin is worth a try

You may try

1. Check for medications and herbs that interfere with statin metabolism (e.g., St. John's Wort)
2. A different statin at a lower dose. Prava and fluva have the fewest reported myalgias. Of all statins, extended-release fluva has perhaps the lowest rate of myalgias. Consider pitava, because it is only marginally metabolized through CYP450 mechanism.
3. A very low dose of rosuva. Low as in 2.5 mg daily or even 1 mg daily or either of those every other day
4. Red yeast rice at 1,800 mg/day (note: rhabomyolysis has occurred with red yeast rice, because the active ingredient in red yeast rice is naturally occurring lova)
5. Ensure adequate vitamin D stores; check 25 OH vitamin D
6. And, as the last best try: stop the statins for 6 weeks while you get the vitamin D level to normal and replenish with 200 mg of coenzyme Q10. Then restart a low dose of a different statin every other day for a month and increase until tolerance or full dose

Step 2 if truly statin intolerant

1. Start sterols and stanols, a diet that strictly limits saturated and trans-fats and exogenous cholesterol, and includes soluble fibers
2. If statins fail, start ezetimibe 10 or colesevelam 6 tabs daily

Step 3. If more LDL-C lowering required, combine colesevelam and the ezetimibe with the diet changes

Chapter 12

A Health-promoting Lifestyle

Some people decide to choose good health, while others actually choose bad health. Everyday choices promote either good or bad health. Oatmeal or a donut. Stairs or escalator. Tuna sandwich with salad or double bacon cheeseburger with fries. These little choices add up to good health or disease and disability.

The outcome differences are huge: healthy people live 14 years longer and in better health than people who consistently make unhealthy choices. Healthy people live seven years longer than average people, while those who choose bad health also chose more disability, more chronic disease, and an early death. They choose disease by smoking or being sedentary or making poor food choices, or being obese. And they die 14 years before the people who made healthy choices.

Dr. Cosgrove, CEO of the Cleveland Clinic says, "Three things—smoking, diet, and lack of exercise—cause 40% of premature deaths in the US. They contribute 70% of the chronic diseases, things like emphysema and heart disease. And 75% of the cost of health care." (Colvin, G. *Fortune Magazine,* March 1, 2010)

The health habits of long-lived people, those with minimal disease or disability, are quite simple and based very much on common sense. Good health does not require Spandex and tofu. Good health requires only not smoking, a sensible and balanced diet of non-processed foods, daily physical activity, and not being obese. Preferably life-long. Great health requires only a little more.

Earlier we talked about both elevated cholesterol and inflammation causing heart disease. So far, we have devoted the book to lowering LDL-C. How do we lower inflammation? Well, statins lower inflammation. Not smoking lowers inflammation. Having a normal weight lowers inflammation. Controlling hypertension lowers inflammation. Daily activity (> the equivalent of 30 minutes of brisk walking) lowers inflammation. Eating a Mediterranean-type diet lowers inflammation. Having a normal blood sugar lowers inflammation. Wow, the AHA's Simple Seven lower inflammation.

Little of our most powerful medical care is as powerful and beneficial as a healthy lifestyle. An unhealthy lifestyle makes treatment nearly futile. Some patients can and do eat and sit their way to an early grave despite our best efforts at medical treatment.

As life expectancy has increased over the past century, we are no longer dying in childhood or young adulthood from infections. Rather we are now living long enough to develop and die from chronic diseases that are the direct result of our lifestyle choices.

As the saying goes, "The older you are, the healthier you have been." With few exceptions, genetics account for no more than 30% of a person's health. Even at that, a good physician will use a bad family history as an important clue to start aggressive prevention measures before the disease develops.

Let's look again at the healthy version of American Heart's Simple Seven:

1. Do not smoke.
2. Maintain a healthy weight.
3. Be active.
4. Eat a healthy diet.

5. Know and treat your blood pressure to recommended levels.
6. Know and treat your cholesterols to normal levels.
7. Keep your blood sugar normal.

As discussed in Chapter 1, the INTERHEART study identified nine attributes that account for over 90% of heart disease. Two of these are best treated with medication (elevated LDL and hypertension), and one requires public health and economic intervention (psycho-social factors). Otherwise, heart disease is associated with the lifestyle choices: whether to smoke, whether to be obese, eat a poor diet, get regular activity, or drink alcohol in moderation.

Most of the data correlating lifestyle choices with premature heart disease are observational and epidemiologic. These studies are complicated by confounding variables because people who engage in daily exercise are also likely to eat a heart-healthy diet, to not smoke, and to be normal weight.

The data from multiple observational and epidemiologic studies are consistent with each other and help science identify optimal lifestyles that promote good health and minimal risk of disease. A health-promoting and cardiovascular-disease-minimizing lifestyle consists of incorporating exercise and activity into each day; consistently eating good proteins, good carbohydrates, and good fats; no tobacco; not being obese or abusing alcohol.

Tobacco

Wow, is a tobacco section necessary?

Smoking causes premature heart disease and cancer. Smoking kills. Mountains of scientific proof, going all the way back to the great studies of Doll and Peto in the 1950s on survival differences in British physicians by smoking status.

End of discussion.

Next topic, please.

Exercise and physical activity

Healthy people, those with a low risk of cardiovascular disease, make being active a routine part of their daily activities. Unhealthy people, those with a high risk of cardiovascular disease, shun physical activity and exercise.

This distinction is important because the real health risks—and almost doubling of mortality—arise when people are sedentary. Nearly two thirds of all Americans are either sedentary or do so little activity that it does not count. A third of Americans are sedentary and do no, none, zip physical activity; another third get so little activity that it does not count—being active only 10 minutes most days of the week or active 30 minutes once or twice a week; and only a scant third of people get more activity that 30 minutes of walking briskly most days of the week.

The health benefits start as soon as people begin to walk as little as 30 minutes five days a week. Getting a sedentary person to walk 30 minutes every day provides a bigger health gain than telling a regular walker to train for a marathon. The benefit is even greater if more activity is also added throughout the day (e.g., a brisk 30-minute walk plus stairs instead of the escalator, walking quickly around the block on the way to lunch, actively playing ball with the kids in the evening, or doing real gardening).

Multiple studies show that cardiovascular mortality decreases 20% to 30% in those who do any type of physical activity that burns 2,000 kcal per week. (Lee IM, Paffanbarger RS *JAMA* 1995; 273: 1179–1184) This works out to only 150 minutes of activity (think brisk walking) per week, or 30 minutes five days a week. This benefit is seen in both men and women; in young, middle-aged, and elderly; in sedentary people who start to exercise; in both primary and secondary cardiovascular prevention; and in known diabetics.

Exercise is beneficial and improves the known cardiovascular risk factors. Exercise improves the lipid profile by lowering triglycerides and increasing HDL, lowers blood pressure, decreases insulin resistance and abdominal adiposity thus preventing type 2 diabetes, reduces inflammatory markers, and improves endothelial function.

Chart 9 Mortality in 16,000 veterans by time on a treadmill at year 0 of the study (adapted from Kokkinos P et al., "Exercise Capacity in Black and White Men" *Circulation.* 2008; 117: 614–622)

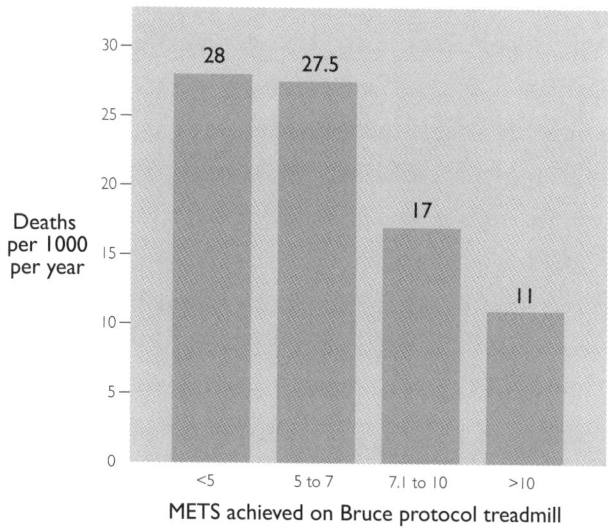

The recommendations from almost everyone—the Centers for Disease Control, the National Institutes of Health, the US Surgeon General, the American Heart Association, the College of Sports Medicine, the American Diabetes Association, and the American Cancer Society—state that everyone should get a minimum of 30 minutes of physical activity most days of the week—and more, or the addition of vigorous exercise or strength training, is even better.

Diet

The foods we choose to eat (or not to eat) directly impact our health, both for better or worse.

A diet that promotes premature disease

What makes up a healthy diet? Debate and confusion surround this question. But there is little disagreement about what constitutes an unhealthy diet.

Few people have trouble identifying a disease-causing diet. Tragically, this is a diet that too many people eat without a second thought. This diet actually promotes disease. It is filled with highly processed, nutritionally deficient, calorie-dense food, often eaten on the run. It leads to obesity, type 2 diabetes, premature heart disease, and, arguably, some cancers.

Even our national "good diet" messages often have unintended consequences. Telling Americans to "eat less fat and more carbohydrates" was an invitation for disaster. What the authorities really meant was "eat less saturated and trans-fats" and more whole grains, but the American public heard "if you eat less fat, you can eat all of the refined carbohydrates such as pretzels and 'fat-free' ice cream you want."

Unfortunately, this unhealthy diet looks much like what most of the advanced and economically advantaged world eats today: breakfast is a bagel, a donut (or three), or processed and sugared cereals and a soda; a mid-morning snack is another donut and a soda; lunch is a fast-food taco or Caesar chicken wrap with fries and a soda; an afternoon snack is chips or a candy bar and a soda; and dinner is a frozen pizza and a soda followed by too many cookies while watching television.

Q: How do you fatten a cow?
A: Put it in a pen where it has minimal movement and feed it corn.

Q: How do you fatten an American male?
A: Put him in a recliner, turn on Sunday football, and feed him chips and beer or soda.

The medical consequences of this Western diet are well-known. Numerous studies document the link between diets high in both trans- and saturated fats and cardiovascular disease. The worst fats are the trans-fats because they raise both LDL-C and lower HDL-C. When people replaced fats, they ate highly processed carbohydrates: think sugar and white flour. Some experts believe that the all-too-common "low-fat products" contribute directly to the national pandemic of diabesity.

This all-too-common Western diet provides a plethora of highly refined, nutritionally deficient, calorie-dense products made from white flours, saturated and trans-fats, sugars, salt, and enough chemicals to start a small factory. And causes enough disease to keep cardiologists and endocrinologists busy for years.

Table 34 Comparison of a typical Western and optimal diet

	Typical Western	Optimal or prudent
Breakfast	Bagel with cream cheese	Oatmeal with berries and OJ
Lunch	Frozen microwave pizza with soda	Tuna salad on dark lettuce with other veggies
Snack	16-ounce latte with a 600 calorie cookie	Grapes and walnuts
Dinner	12-ounce rib eye steak, French fries, soda	6 ounce salmon, green beans, sweet potato
Evening snack	Large bag of cookies and ice cream	A pear, one small cookie and a cup of tea
Eating place	Car, desk at work, or while watching television	Home dining table with family or café with friends

A diet that promotes good health

A health-promoting diet is an array of different foods that work synergistically to maximize good cellular and biochemical health, minimize wide swings of blood sugar and insulin, reduce inflammation, and regulate fatty acid and lipid production. These foods are eaten mindfully at meal-time (read: at the dining table with family or friends, not in a car or while watching television).

A health-promoting diet is not just eating a couple of the recently identified "super foods." Sure, blue berries, spinach, and salmon are excellent foods. But an occasional blueberry smoothie and piece of salmon cannot do much if the rest of the week is donuts and frozen pizza.

Nor is a health-promoting diet achieved only with supplements. Does anyone really know what phytochemicals are in an orange? A wheat kernel? Sure, we think we are getting vitamin C when we eat an orange or vitamin E when we eat wheat germ. But we are undoubtedly also eating 400 other phytochemicals, and one of them, or more likely a combination of them, are acting synergistically to promote good health.

A health-promoting diet means eating good proteins, good carbohydrates (e.g., whole grains), healthy fats and oils, and a wide variety of colorful fruits and vegetables.

The American Heart Association recently released their national goals for cardiovascular health promotion and disease reduction. (*Circulation,* 2010; 121: 586–613)

Table 35 The 2010 dietary goals of the American Heart Association

Primary dietary goals	▸ fruits and veggies	▸ ≥ 4.5 cups per day
	▸ fiber-rich foods	▸ ≥ 3 one-ounce servings per day
	▸ oily fish	▸ ≥ 2 3.5-ounce servings per week
	▸ sodium	▸ < 1,500 mg per day
	▸ sugar-sweetened beverages	▸ < 36 ounces per week
Secondary dietary goals	▸ nuts, seeds, and legumes	▸ ≥ 4 servings of per week
	▸ processed meat	▸ ≤ 2 servings of per week
	▸ saturated fat	▸ < 7% of total energy intake

A few food notes on the AHA's 2010 recommendations:

- Fruits and veggies are self-explanatory. The average American eats 1.6 servings of fruits and veggies a day. *(http://www.cdc.gov/mmwr/preview/mmwrhtml/mm5610a2.htm)*
- Normal-weight people were more likely to eat fruits and veggies than overweight or obese people, who ate the fewest.

  Here is how to easily eat nine one-half-cup servings a day: breakfast is OJ (1 serving) and berries or banana (2) on oatmeal; lunch is soup or half sandwich with a dark green leafy salad with tomato, cucumber, beets (3, 4, 5); afternoon snack is an apple (6); dinner is a fish or chicken with a sweet potato (7) and green beans (8); dessert is blueberry (9) pie (just don't eat the crust).

- The AHA defines a "high fiber food" as 1 gram of fiber per 10 calories because many foods are promoted as "whole grain" when, in reality, they only contain a smidgeon of whole grain. As a start, a "fiber-rich" slice of bread should provide at least 3 grams of fiber.
- Oily fish does not mean deep fried. An oily fish is a fish that is high in the cardio-protective omega-3s. This means ocean fish such as salmon, tuna, or sardines, or the fresh- and cold-water trout. It does not mean tilapia or catfish, who are raised in a fish farm in Mississippi.
- The average American eats 3,500 mg of sodium every day. Eighty percent of that amount is in processed or store-bought food—think hot dogs, chips, soups, salsas, and French fries.
- Thirty-six-ounces of sweetened soda a week is only three 12-ounce cans of soda or sweetened tea. Not much—many people have 36 ounces or more each day.
- In a 2,000 cal diet, 7% is 140 calories, so that is not much saturated fat. One tablespoon of butter is 68 calories of saturated fat, a cup of 2% milk is 40 calories of saturated fat, a hot dog is 140 calories of fat, and five Oreo cookies is 90 grams of fat.

An optimal diet

An optimal and prudent diet consists of minimal trans-fats; processed foods, salt, and sugared drinks and snacks. This prudent diet has modest amounts of red meat; at least five colorful fruits and veggies every day, along with a serving or two of whole grains or beans; ocean fish at least twice a week; nuts frequently; and olive or polyunsaturated oils as the primary fat. Perhaps the best dietary advice would be that everyone, both men and women, take cooking classes so they better understand exactly how much of what they are eating.

This prudent or optimal diet is high in phytochemicals, especially if it includes a wide variety of colorful fruits and veggies—for example, apples, grapes, kiwi, melons, peaches, oranges, plums, figs, broccoli, dark lettuces, green beans, beets, asparagus, tomatoes, yams, peppers, carrots, and persimmons.

A prudent diet includes ocean fish at least twice a week. This ensures an adequate intake of omega-3 fats EPA and DHA. Multiple studies document the benefits of omega-3 fats found in deep water ocean fish. The American Heart Association suggests that all adults eat two servings of ocean fish every week, or take 500 mg of omega-3 EPA + DHA daily.

This prudent diet that we have outlined above is consistent with what many people call a "Mediterranean diet." Several interesting studies support eating a Mediterranean diet. Perhaps because a Mediterranean diet both proscribes foods and substances (read trans-fats because it is not really a food, it is a chemical) known to cause cardiovascular disease and prescribes foods known to be cardio-protective (omega-3 fats, fruits, veggies, nuts, cereals, and some alcohol).

The famous 1999 Lyon Heart Study studied 600 patients who had suffered one heart attack and were placed on either whatever their cardiologist considered a heart-prudent diet or something close to a Mediterranean modification of the AHA diet. This "experimental Mediterranean diet" consisted of more fish; more green vegetables including root veggies; fruit every day; more bread; a substitution of poultry for red meat; an α-linolenic acid-enriched margarine in place of cream and butter; and the use of canola or olive oil for both salads and food preparation. The results are shown in the following chart, clearly demonstrating the benefit of a Mediterranean diet.

Chart 10 Event-free survival for MI or death adapted from Lyon Heart Study (adapted from Lorgeril et al. *Circ* 1999; 99: 779–785)

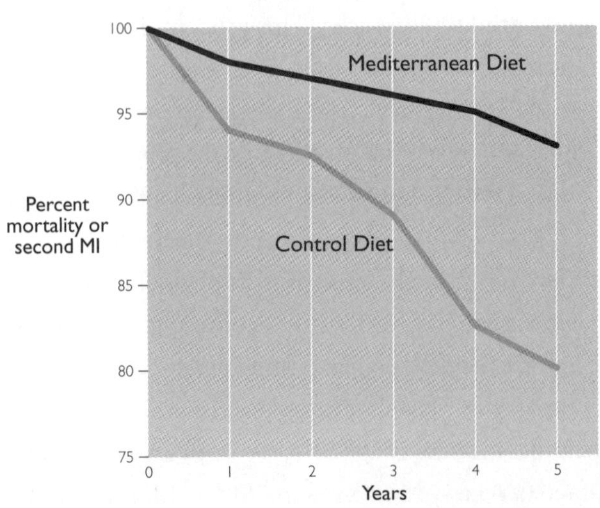

Note that the Lyon Heart Study used a margarine that contained α-linolenic acid (ALA). ALA is found naturally in some nuts and vegetables oils.

Dietary treatment of hypertriglyceridemia

Very high levels of triglycerides require strict lifestyle and dietary management. These dietary guidelines are different from dietary changes for control of total- and LDL-C because they restrict all fat consumption. Aerobic exercise and even modest weight loss often help lower triglycerides. If the triglycerides exceed 1,000, a diet that lowers total fat to < 10% of total calories usually drops the triglycerides by half. Importantly, triglyceride levels are determined by the total amount of simple carbohydrates and fat in the diet, but not by the type of fat.

The reasons for fat restriction are three-fold: fat restriction (1) reduces both chylomicrons and VLDL-P production, (2) reduces the burden of circulating triglycerides on the LPL, and (3) causes weight loss, which eventually slows FFA production and reduces insulin resistance. Dietary management of hypertriglyceridemia also requires eating complex carbohydrates instead of simple carbohydrates (oatmeal instead of a bagel), avoiding fructose found in most sodas and fruit drinks, and avoiding alcohol. Perhaps the most effective diet to lower triglycerides is a very low carb (e.g., 50 gram) diet.

Dietary treatment of a low HDL-C

On the other hand, some patients with a low HDL-C and possibly mildly elevated triglyceride may be eating a very low-fat diet. These patients will benefit from the addition of healthy mono- and poly-unsaturated fats to their diets.

Additional dietary ways to lower LDL-C

The American Heart Association's proposed diet is designed to improve lipids and reduce cardiovascular disease.

The addition of plant sterols and stanols can result in even more LDL-C lowering. These compete with cholesterol for absorption by gut enzyme

NPC1L1. They effectively reduce the absorption of cholesterol by 65%, which lowers the plasma LDL-C by 5% to 10%. The average person eats 150 to 400 mg of plant sterols and 20 to 50 mg of plant stanols a day; the therapeutic dose of plant sterols necessary to lower LDL-C is 2,000 mg a day. We tell our patients to buy stanols and sterols in a pill form (e.g., CholestOff).

Red rice yeast is another non-FDA-approved dietary addition that can lower LDL-C. It contains a low dose of a naturally produced lovastatin. Although red rice yeast has been associated with myalgias and even with rhabdomyolysis, it is generally very well-tolerated. Doses of 1,800 to 2,400 mg daily can lower LDL-C by 10%. As a non-FDA-approved supplement, the potency and purity of this product is not assured.

A day to make the Heart Association happy

Let's use the AHA's 2010 recommendations to plan a day. Breakfast is a glass of OJ, oatmeal or a bowl of whole grain cereal (e.g., shredded wheat or Wheaties) with raisins or berries on top, or maybe an English muffin with a sterol-enriched margarine and the jam from the farmer's market. This meal is eaten at the table with your family. You are at two colorful fruits and either one or two servings of fiber-rich foods.

Drive to work, but park a half mile away and walk briskly to the office.

With a group of friends from work, you go to the neighborhood café, where you sit outside in the sun. Lunch is bean and ham soup (your legume for the day) and a salad of dark leafy greens with tomato, cucumber, and sunflower seeds topped with olive oil and vinegar. The large salad got you 3 more colorful veggies, some seeds, and olive oil.

Afternoon snack is classic trail mix (granola, nuts, raisins, and M&Ms) with water. More seeds, some chocolate.

On the way home, you walk the half mile back to your car. Then stop at the club for 15 minutes of elliptical and 30 minutes of various yoga sun salutations.

Dinner is a glass of wine (all right, two glasses, but not more than three), grilled salmon with grilled asparagus and a sweet potato. Dessert is blackberry pie—just eat the filling and leave the crust. An oily fish with omega-3s, and two more veggies (yam and broccoli). Plus the yam is filled with fiber.

At the end of this day, you ate 8 servings of colorful fruits and veggies, more than four servings of fiber-rich foods, one oily fish, lots of nuts, seeds, and legumes; minimal sodium, some olive and sunflower oil, nearly no saturated fat, and no processed foods. And some sterols. Not bad. Plus, you walked more than a mile and exercised vigorously for 45 minutes.

Selected Studies with Notes

THE FOLLOWING STUDIES are an introduction to some of the important lipid studies. Any review of studies is quickly complicated and compromised because of second look studies or a reanalysis of the data. We have tried to stick with the initial purpose of the study with our comments and notes aimed specifically at our target audience: the provider in the trenches.

As you review the studies remember that patients in the early studies usually had very high cholesterol values, where the observed benefit is expected to be large.

The abbreviation DBPCR means "double-blind, placebo-controlled, randomized."

Table 36 First studies to show benefit of lower lipids

LRC-CPPT	1973 to 1984	▸ BAS or placebo ▸ At entry LDL> 190, asymptomatic men with hypercholesterolemia ▸ LDL ↓ by 13%, ▸ CHD death or nonfatal MI ↓ 19% ▸ Overall mortality ↓ 7% ▸ 19% ↓ CHD death and/or MI
Helsinki Heart Study	1987	▸ Gemfibrozil or placebo ▸ Asymptomatic men with non-HDL-C ≥ 200 ▸ LDL ↓ 11% HDL ↑ 11% ▸ CAD endpoints ↓ 34% ▸ Greatest benefit when initial TG high and HDL low ▸ If LDL/HDL > 5.0 and TG > 200, risk fell by 71% ▸ The 22% ↓ in end points was seen with a 6% ↑ in HDL and a 31% ↓ in TG but no change in LDL

Table 37 First studies to show benefit of statins

4S	1994	▶ Primary and secondary study ▶ DBRPC ▶ Starting TC was 213 to 309 ▶ 20 mg of Simva or placebo ▶ Study goal was TC 116 to 200 ▶ 36% decrease in LDL ▶ 30% reduction in overall mortality, CAD mortality, CAD events
WOSCOPS		▶ Primary prevention of high risk patients ▶ Prava 40 or placebo ▶ LDL-C down by 20% ▶ CAD and CAD deaths down by 31%
CARE		▶ Cholesterol and Recurrent Events Trial ▶ Secondary prevention, history of MI required ▶ Starting LDL-C averaged 139 ▶ Prava 40 or placebo ▶ LDL down by 32% to 97 ▶ CAD recurrence and mortality down by 24%
LIPID		▶ Long-term intervention with Prava in Ischemic Disease ▶ Secondary prevention, history of MI or angina ▶ Prava 40 or placebo ▶ Starting TC 155 to 270 ▶ CAD and all-cause mortality down 24% ▶ Risk for stroke down 19%
AFCAPS/ TexCAPS		▶ Primary prevention ▶ Starting TC 220 ▶ Lova 20 or placebo ▶ First trial to show benefit of statins in patients with average TC and LDL and below average HDL ▶ LDL down by 25% ▶ First CAD event down by 37%

Table 38 Benefit in high-risk primary prevention

HPS	1994 to 2001	▸ First study to look at high risk sub groups 20,000 pts (women, elderly, those with below average LDL-C) ▸ Starting LDL-C 130, HDL-C 41, and TG 181 ▸ Secondary or high risk pts ▸ Simva and/or anti-oxidants or placebo ▸ 30% improvement in mortality and events regardless of LDL at start even those with LDL < 100 at start ▸ No increase mortality statin versus placebo for non-CAD deaths ▸ Anti-oxidants made results worse ▸ HPS formed basis for 2004 Update of ATP III recommending LDL target of < 100 and optional < 70

Table 39 Benefit of intensive versus standard therapy in secondary prevention and ACS

MIRACL	2004	▸ Myocardial Ischemia Reduction through Cholesterol Lowering ▸ Intensive therapy immediately following ACS ▸ Atorva 80 or placebo ▸ At end of 16 weeks, there was a 16% reduction in events ▸ LDL fell from 124 to 72
TNT	2005	▸ Secondary study ▸ Stable CAD ▸ Atorva 10 versus 80 in patients with LD: < 130 ▸ Rx LDLs were 101 and 72 ▸ Intensive Rx group had lower mortality ▸ End point was next CV event or death ▸ Higher statin more beneficial than lower in both healthy and diabetic ▸ all cause mortality ↓ ▸ mortality in elderly ↓ ▸ hosp for heart failure ↓ ▸ rate of ↑ LFT ↑
PROVE-IT		▸ Enrolled pts within 10 days of an MI ▸ Prava 40 versus atorva 80 ▸ Starting LDL 106, prava 95, atorva to 62 ▸ RR 22% ▸ Lowering LDL down to 40 had better outcomes than LDL at 60 with no increase in non-CAD adverse events

PROVE-IT-TIMI 22		▸ Atorva 80 versus prava 20 or 40 w/Ii 10 days of coronary event ▸ After 2 years, a 16% reduction with intensive Rx ▸ The benefit was seen with 30 days of starting Rx ▸ But hepatic events 3.3% with intensive Rx versus 1.1% with prava 20 or 40 ▸ Intensive Rx group had a 3.9% ARR and 16% RRR in all cause mortality, MI, angina ▸ Rates of stroke did NOT differ between the two groups ▸ LFT ↑ ▸ Angina requiring hosp ↓ ▸ Revascularization ↓ ▸ More benefit with LDL > 125 than when LDL < 125 ▸ Post-hoc analysis, those patients on a statin who achieved a TG < 150 mg/dL had a 27% relative risk reduction in events than did those with a TG of > 150 mg/dL
A to Z		▸ ACS ▸ Simva 40 or 80 versus simva 20 ▸ 11% reduction in CVD death or MI (not significant) ▸ Note 9 of 2500 patients receiving simva 80 developed myopathy and 3 of these developed rhambo.
Courage	2007	▸ Stable angina pts ▸ PCI versus atorva 80 ▸ Results were the same at 5 years
CDP	1975	▸ Secondary prevention trial ▸ Niacin improved lipids and CAD and stroke and total mortality all ↓ ▸ CAD gain not really seen at 5 years, but 11% lower mortality was seen at 9 years
SIHDS		▸ Secondary ▸ Niacin + clofibrate improved lipids and ↓CAD
CLAS		▸ Secondary ▸ BAS = niacin ▸ Improved lipids, ↓progression and ↑regression ▸ Benefit limited to those with TG > 133 and most pronounced in those whose TG fell by > 30% ▸ BAS alone or with niacin or lova lowers CHD risk by 58% and enhances regression by 16%

SAFARI		▸ Safety of statin and fenofibrate ▸ No cases of rhabdomyolysis
Explorer		▸ Secondary study ▸ Treatment group had LDL of 190 to 250, G < 450 ▸ Ezetimibe + rosuva 40 versus rosuva 40 ▸ Endpoint was meeting ATP goal ▸ Of combo patients, 94% reached target LDL of 100 and 79% reached target of 70—higher than the rosuva alone
MARS		▸ Monitored Atherosclerosis Regression Study ▸ Lova versus placebo ▸ ↓ LDL-c, Apo B, and VLDL-c ▸ HDL and Lp(a) no change
COMBOS		▸ Statin + POM3 ▸ More patients reached non-HDL goals by TG ↓ 29% and LDL ↑ 3%, but Apo B ↓ 8%, HDL only ↑ 2%

Table 40 Intravascular ultrasound studies

REVERSAL		▸ Subjects had luminal irregularities 20% to 50%, but no occlusion and an LDL-C 125 to 210 ▸ Atorva 80 versus prava 40 ▸ IVUS used in study results ▸ Progression was halted by atorva 80 but progressed 2.6% with prava 40
ASTEROID		▸ Rosuva 40 ▸ Pts had CAD and LDL-C of 130 ▸ Rx reduced LDL-C to 60 and HDL-C rose 15% ▸ More aggressive therapy caused atheroma regression

Table 41 Study to show that statin Rx in patients with stroke or TIA but no CAD can reduce second event

SPARCL		▸ LDL down ▸ 16% reduction in second stroke ▸ 35% reduction in major CAD ▸ Neither total or LDL cholesterol before or after Rx impacted hemorrhagic stroke risk
HPS		▸ See Table 35 above

Table 42 Benefit of fish oil

GISSI-Prevenzione		▸ POM3 ↓ overall mortality, CV mortality, sudden death ▸ Did not reduce stroke
DART		▸ Secondary study ▸ Those eating fatty fish had 29% lower over-all mortality
JELLIS		▸ Low dose statin + fish oil versus low dose statin ▸ 24% reduction in any major CAD event regardless of TG levels ▸ NNT to prevent one death or CAD hospitalization over 4 years = 44

Table 43 Statins plus niacin

HATS	2001	▸ Angiography study of % change in stenosis ▸ Patients had angio proven CAD and low HDL (< 35 men, 40 women) and LDL < 140 ▸ Statin + niacin versus placebo ▸ Results worsened with anti-oxidants ▸ Secondary study showing CHD events declined markedly 60% to 90% with simva + niacin compared to none ▸ Statin + niacin showed regression (but those on statin + niacin + anti-oxidants progressed) ▸ Rx combo ↑ HDL, VLDL ↓
ARBITER 2		▸ Adding ER Niacin 1000 to statin (all pts on a statin at start) ▸ CIMT ▸ Niacin + statin reduced CIMT progression ▸ Adding niacin ^ HDL 21% (40 to 47) ▸ Less but still some benefit in type 2 DM and MET-S ▸ Conclusion: ^ HDL responsible for benefit
ARBITER 3		▸ 1 tear extension ▸ Now started to see regression in both placebo + ERN and statin + ERN although statin + ERN had more progression
AIM-HIGH	ongoing	▸ Looking at benefits of statin versus statin + niacin

Table 44 Fibrate studies (Helsinki, VA HIT, FIELD)

FIELD	2005	▸ Largest study of CV events in diabetics (7500 primary and 2000 secondary prevention) ▸ Patients had DM, but normal lipids, ▸ Fenofibrate 200 mg/d ▸ Study confounded by statin drop-ins ▸ No cases of rhabdomyolysis ▸ With combo, TG, LDL, non-HDL all ↓ and HDL ↑compared to monotherapy ▸ With combo, CK → no change ▸ With combo LFT ↑ ▸ 11% to 20% improvement in CAD and CHD deaths with Rx in primary but not secondary prevention ▸ Again, biggest effect if high TG and low HDL
Helsinki heart	1987	▸ Primary study ▸ LDL ↓ 11% HDL ↑ 11% ▸ CAD endpoints ↓ 34% ▸ Greatest benefit when initial TG high and HDL low ▸ If LDL/HDL > 5.0 and TG > 200, risk fell by 71%
VA HIT	1999	▸ Secondary study ▸ Gemfibrozil lowered events in people with low HDL ▸ LDL no change ▸ TG ↓ 31% ▸ HDL ↑ 6%—the best predictor of success in the trial ▸ MI or nonfatal CHD ↓ 22% ▸ Stoke ↓ 24%
DAIS		▸ Diabetes atherosclerosis intervention study ▸ Fenofibrate versus placebo ▸ Angiographic study ▸ LDL-P ↑ with fenofibrate ▸ Fewer CHD events and smaller decrease in coronary artery diameter

Table 45 Statins lower hsCRP and mortality

JUPITER	2008	▸ 17,000 subjects with LDL-C < 130 and hsCRP > 2.0 ▸ Compared placebo to rosuva 20 ▸ End point of MI, stroke, revascularization, unstable angina, or death from CV event ▸ Trial stopped after 1.9 years because rosuva lowered events by 56% ▸ On-treatment LDL-C fell by 50% and hsCRP fell by 37% ▸ On-treatment LDL-C ranged from 42 to 70

Table 46 Enzymes important in lipid biology

ACAT	▸ acyl-CoA cholestserol acyl transferase
ABCA-1	▸ ATP-binding cassette transporter ▸ Absent in Tangier disease so cholesterol concentrations build in both lymphatic (e.g., spleen and tonsils) and vascular tissues
ABCG-1	▸ Transport of cholesterol within macrophages and in foam cell formation to the nascent HDL-P
Adipokines	▸ Proteins secreted by adipocytes ▸ Include a range of enzymes including cytokines, growth factors, enzymes, hormones ▸ Functions: appetite and energy balance, immunity, insulin sensitivity, angiogenesis, inflammation, acute phase response
Adiponectin	▸ Secreted by adipocytes ▸ Higher levels associated with lower risk of CAD ▸ Lower levels in obese people
Apo A-I	▸ Major protein of HDL ▸ 1 to 4 copies of apo A-1 on each HDL-P ▸ Modulates activity of LCAT ▸ Produced in liver and jejunum ▸ Secreted into blood either as free A-I or attached to chylomicron and VLDL
Apo A-II	▸ Major protein of HDL ▸ Activates hepatic lipase
Apo A-IV	▸ Secreted by intestine and association with chylomicron formation ▸ May control food intake in hypothalamus
Apo B	▸ The apo-lipoprotein involved with chylomicron (apo B-48); and VLDL, IDL, and LDL apo B-100 ▸ The protein factor recognized by hepatic LDL-R (LDL-Receptors, which are necessary for the removal of LDL)

Apo B-48	▸ Produced in intestine for chylomicron synthesis and transport of triglycerides
Apo B-100	▸ Made in liver ▸ Binds to hepatic LDL-R ▸ Transport of TG and CE
Apo C-I	▸ Synthesized in liver and activates LCAT and LPL
APo C-II	▸ Synthesized in liver and ▸ activates LCAT and ▸ obligate co-factor for LPL
APo C-III	▸ Synthesized in liver and inhibits LPL ▸ Modulates uptake of TG-rich particles by LRP
Apo E	▸ Synthesized in liver, main function is to transport cholesterol ▸ 2/2 Type III Dysbetalipoproteinemia and protects against CAD and stroke ▸ 3/3 most common ▸ 4/4 ▸ Greatest risk for CVD ▸ Increased risk of Alzheimer's ▸ Smoking increases CVD risk most
Apo B-48	▸ B protein on chylomicrons ▸ Produced in jejunum ▸ Lacks ability to bind with LDL-R
Apo B-100	▸ B protein on VLDL, IDL, LDL ▸ Binds to LDL-R
CETP	▸ cholesteryl ester transfer protein ▸ Is induced by high-fat and high-cholesterol diet ▸ Exercise decreases CETP activity ▸ High plasma levels of CETP are associated with low levels of HDL and a TG/HDL ratio > 3.8
DGAT2	▸ Diglyceride acyltransferase
Endothelial lipase	▸ The second step of hydrolysis of HDL ▸ HDL often made so small after EL activity that it is excreted in urine

FXR	▸ Farnesoid X receptor
	▸ A nuclear receptor that regulates gene expression in response to bile acids
	▸ Induces apo C-II transcription
	▸ Increased by fibrates and PPAR
	▸ FXR expression has hypo-triglyceridemic effects by:
	  ▸ Inducing PPAR-α expression
	  ▸ Modulating lipoprotein lipase
	  ▸ Activation of FXR inhibits sterol regulatory binding element protein-1C (SREB-1c) which is mediated through the short heterodimer protein (SHP) negative effect on LXR

Ghrelin	▸ Produced in stomach ▸ Stimulates growth hormone ▸ Increases hunger and food intake, but reduces fat utilization in adipocytes ▸ Blood levels decrease after eating and increase during a fast
Hepatic Lipase	▸ Endothelial anchored enzyme ▸ Responsible for hydrolysis of TG and phospholipids from IDL and HDL ▸ Activated by apo B
HDL	▸ Functions of HDL: RCT and cellular cholesterol efflux, anti-inflammatory, anti-oxidant, anti-infectious, anti-apoptotic, anti-thrombotic (inhibits endothelial cell adhesion and MCP-1), vasoldilatory, endothelial repair, inhibits up-regulation of ICAM-1 and VCAM-1i, inhibits LDL oxidations, up-regulates PGI2 (anti-coagulant) ▸ Is the Lp that delivers cholesterol to steroidogenic organs
HDL-2	▸ Rich in CE, made from HDL-2
HDL-3	▸ Scavenges free cholesterol from blood vessels, esterifies cholesterol via LCAT and apo A-1
Inflammatory transcription factors	▸ Nf-KB, HIF-1, AP-1
LCAT	▸ Lecithin-cholesterol acyltransferase ▸ Converts free cholesterol to cholesterol ester ▸ Deficiency causes low HDL and fish eye disease

LDL-R	▸ LDL-Receptors on the surface of the liver that attach to apo B and apo E of VLDL-P, IDL-P, and LDL-P. This removes the particles from circulation and lowers the systemic LDL-C and triglyceride and increases the hepatic level of cholesterol
Leptin	▸ Secreted from adipocytes, enters brain to regulate feeding
LPL	▸ Lipoprotein lipase ▸ Cleaves fatty acids from triacylglycerol within lipoproteins releasing fatty acids ▸ Associated with endothelium ▸ Major source of fatty acids for energy for heart and skeletal muscle
Lp-PLA2	▸ Lipoprotein-associated phospholipase A2 ▸ Elevated levels imply active vascular disease ▸ Not correlated with other markers of inflammation like CRP so has an independent role in inflammation
LXR	▸ Liver X receptor ▸ Nuclear receptors that are sensitive to cholesterol ▸ High cholesterol levels in cell prompt LXR to start process to activate enzymes to remove cholesterol ▸ Regulate cytokines, suppress hepatic glucose production
MMP	▸ Proteolytic enzyme associated with plaque rupture
MTP	▸ Microsomal transfer protein ▸ In liver ▸ Assembles TG and CE with apo B and E and phospholipid to make VLDL
NF-K β	▸ Regulates the expression of inflammatory molecules including VCAM and ICAM
NPC1L1	▸ Niemann-Pick C1-Like 1 ▸ Cholesterol and other (phyto)sterols from gut into systemic circulation ▸ Site where ezetimibe works ▸ Ezetimibe normally lowers LDL by 18%, but 12% of patients lack an NPC1L1 enzyme and their LDL falls 36%; some people have a haplotype where ezetimibe does not work

PAI-1	▸ Inhibitor of fibrinolytic system ▸ ^ PAI-1 associated with increased risk of MI
PPAR α	▸ Peroxisome proliferator-activated receptor
SREBP	▸ Sterol regulatory element binding protein ▸ SREBP is down-regulated by polyunsaturated fats (e.g., fish oil) which may explain why fish oil lowers TG
SR-B1	▸ Scavenger receptor class B member 1 ▸ Transports cholesterol and CE from HDL ▸ High affinity hepatic receptor that selectively depletes HDL of CEs ▸ Apo A-1 facilitates HDL docking with SR-B1

INDEX

B

C

D

E

M

U

V

W